Clinical Manual of Couples and Family Therapy

by

Gabor I. Keitner, M.D.

Professor of Psychiatry
The Warren Alpert School of Medicine
Brown University/Rhode Island Hospital
Providence, Rhode Island

Alison M. Heru, M.D.

Associate Professor of Psychiatry
University of Colorado Denver
Denver, Colorado

Ira D. Glick, M.D.

Professor of Psychiatry
Stanford University School of Medicine
Stanford, California

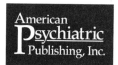

American Psychiatric Publishing, Inc.

Washington, DC
London, England

Note: The authors have worked to ensure that all information in this book is accurate at the time of publication and consistent with general psychiatric and medical standards, and that information concerning drug dosages, schedules, and routes of administration is accurate at the time of publication and consistent with standards set by the U.S. Food and Drug Administration and the general medical community. As medical research and practice continue to advance, however, therapeutic standards may change. Moreover, specific situations may require a specific therapeutic response not included in this book. For these reasons and because human and mechanical errors sometimes occur, we recommend that readers follow the advice of physicians directly involved in their care or the care of a member of their family.

Books published by American Psychiatric Publishing, Inc., represent the views and opinions of the individual authors and do not necessarily represent the policies and opinions of APPI or the American Psychiatric Association.

Disclosure of interests: The authors have no competing interests or conflicts to declare.

To buy 25–99 copies of this or any other APPI title at a 20% discount, please contact APPI Customer Service at appi@psych.org or 800-368-5777. If you wish to buy 100 or more copies of the same title, please e-mail us at bulksales@psych.org for a price quote.

Copyright © 2010 American Psychiatric Publishing, Inc.
ALL RIGHTS RESERVED

Manufactured in the United States of America on acid-free paper
13   12   11   10   09   5   4   3   2   1
First Edition

Typeset in Adobe's Formata and AGaramond.

American Psychiatric Publishing, Inc.
1000 Wilson Boulevard
Arlington, VA 22209-3901
www.appi.org

Library of Congress Cataloging-in-Publication Data
Keitner, Gabor I., 1947-
  Clinical manual of couples and family therapy / by Gabor I. Keitner, Alison Margaret Heru, Ira D. Glick.
    p. ; cm.
  Includes bibliographical references and index.
  ISBN 978-1-58562-290-0 (alk. paper)
  1. Family psychotherapy. 2. Marital psychotherapy. I. Heru, Alison M., 1953- II. Glick, Ira D., 1935- III. Title.
  [DNLM: 1. Family Therapy. 2. Couples Therapy. WM 430.5.F2 K27c 2010]
  RC488.5.K445 2010
  616.89'156--dc22
                                                                    2009035107

British Library Cataloguing in Publication Data
A CIP record is available from the British Library.

Contents

DVD Contents

A Guide for Using the Text and DVD

This book was written to provide practical suggestions for conceptualizing psychiatric disorders so as to include family functioning, reasons why such a perspective makes theoretical and practical sense, and a specific method for assessing and treating patients within a family context in addition to treating the families themselves. Because this book is intended to serve as a basic but comprehensive manual for individuals of different training levels and orientations, complex clinical situations and their sequential management regimens have been simplified and compressed. We realize this may be a disadvantage for the more advanced therapist and so have included up-to-date references. The book probably will be most helpful when used with ongoing supervision because most of the case examples and interventions are written in bare-bones detail to make one or two teaching points at a time. For the sake of clarity, some chapters reiterate concepts presented earlier in a different context.

Likewise, a number of chapters are (in our view) too brief to be of value to the experienced family clinician. Here, too, we opted to take the route of maximum breadth, providing appropriate references to flesh out the materials. We believe that the alternative path (i.e., to be less inclusive and provide greater depth) would make this manual too narrow and less useful given the many situations in which family approaches are being used.

We recommend that the beginner read the text sequentially. Each chapter has been written to reinforce concepts introduced in earlier chapters. By reading all of the chapters sequentially, the reader should become more knowledgeable not only about the content reviewed but also about a systematic approach to conceptualizing and dealing with the wide range of problems seen by mental health professionals.

Many of the chapters stand on their own, referencing other relevant chapters in the book as well as the broader professional literature. We are aware of the pressures of time and the large volume of written material with which busy clinicians try to keep up to date. Readers with more limited time, as well as those with experience and expertise with family systems approaches, will benefit from focusing on the specific chapters relevant to their particular interests.

We have included case illustrations throughout the book to relate the concepts described to clinical care and to show a way of operationalizing those concepts while treating common clinical problems. We have also included teaching points at the beginning of each chapter and key points in the body of the chapters. We have done this because the ground that we cover is so broad and can be so confusing to the beginner. The teaching points for each chapter are a summary of the main concepts. The reader can also use them to understand the logic, direction, and end point for each topic. Our terminal objectives include, but are not limited to 1) a general understanding of the underlying theoretical principles and hypotheses behind the family model; 2) an acquaintance with techniques, including an understanding of the advantages and limitations of such techniques; 3) development of an appreciation, through experience, of one's abilities and difficulties in using such techniques; 4) an understanding of how ethnicity, race, gender, and class affect the therapist and family as they work; and 5) an appreciation of the ethical issues involved in all areas of the practice of family intervention.

We have also included a DVD to demonstrate the application of the general approach described in the book, as well as the specific components of assessment and treatment using the McMaster Model of Family Functioning. The DVD shows the assessment of a family presenting with problems related to a long history of depression in the mother. It also shows the first steps in the treatment process, including how to deal with obstacles to improvement.

The DVD is approximately 2½ hours long and is subdivided into 19 scenes, which can be accessed directly. As with the book, the DVD can be watched in its entirety, or the viewer can choose to focus in on specific sections of interest. We suggest that the viewer watch scenes 1–14 continuously to understand the flow of the assessment process. Similarly, the viewer will benefit most by watching the treatment process (scenes 16–18) in its entirety.

The viewer can choose to watch the commentary sections (scene 15 and scene 19) if he or she wants a better understanding of the therapist's thinking about the assessment and treatment process and how these played out with this particular family.

Once the DVD has been viewed as a continuous process, the viewer can return to specific scenes to observe examples of the various components of assessment and treatment. We have also highlighted with **boldface** type areas in the book where particular sections of the DVD illustrate the principles described or where the DVD demonstrates how a particular assessment or intervention can be carried out.

The text and the DVD can be reviewed and used independently but will provide the most useful learning experience when used together interactively.

Acknowledgments

We are grateful for the selfless help provided by a number of colleagues and friends. Nathan B. Epstein, M.D., is the originator of the McMaster Model of Family Functioning and continues to be a role model for ways of integrating biological and psychosocial concepts into case formulation and patient care. Christine E. Ryan, Ph.D., Richard Archambault, Ed.D., Nathan B. Epstein, M.D., and Dwayne Bishop, M.D., members of the Family Research Program at Rhode Island Hospital, have been instrumental in building the foundation for and refining the concepts of the McMaster Model. Marjorie Lederer, M.S.W., and Judi Almeida provided invaluable help in the preparation of this book by reviewing and helping to edit various drafts and ensuring the accuracy of citations. Richard Archambault, Ed.D., Ellen Florin, M.S.W., and Molly Lederer were essential to the preparation of the DVD in agreeing to portray family problems associated with depression. We also want to thank Mark Barone for filming the case illustration and Giovanna Roz of Brown University, who along with her students (Hristo Atanasov, Jerzy Fischer, Grant Kellerman, and Munashe Shumba) did extensive postproduction editing so as to make the DVD as clear and user friendly as possible.

1

Introduction

This book is addressed primarily to physicians, and particularly to psychiatrists. Primary care physicians, pediatricians, gerontologists, and allied mental health professionals will likely also find it useful. One of our goals, however, is to reestablish the role of the psychiatrist as the leader of the team of professionals providing mental health care to patients in need.

The psychiatrist is able to function in this leadership role if he or she is skillful in generating a biopsychosocial formulation of presenting problems and in providing biopsychosocial treatments including pharmacotherapy, psychotherapy, and family interventions. Where such ability or interest in developing broadly based clinical expertise is lacking, psychiatrists are being relegated to supportive roles, most often as providers of psychopharmacological management.

Psychiatrists are in a unique position in the mental health field, with the potential to become skillful in integrating biological, psychological, and social perspectives. They are medically based, trained in psychosocial and interpersonal processes, and able to integrate information from disparate sources.

This broad perspective is consistent with the historical underpinnings of psychiatry. Psychiatric theoreticians over the past hundred years have emphasized biological, psychological, and familial processes. All psychiatrists do not need to become psychotherapists or family therapists. All psychiatrists, however, do need to be proficient in assessing a patient's biological vulnerability to illness, the meaning of that illness to the patient and his or her ways of coping with it, and the social/familial context in which that illness evolves. A comprehensive treatment plan can be designed only with such a thorough understanding of the presenting problem. Even if a psychiatrist chooses to refer a patient to a psychotherapist or family therapist for more extensive therapy work, the psychiatrist still needs to know which kind of therapy is most likely to be helpful, be able to evaluate the quality and appropriateness of the therapies, and, most importantly, be able to integrate the therapy work into the comprehensive treatment plan.

This book presents a conceptual framework for engaging families of patients with psychiatric symptoms, problems, and disorders. We outline family therapy skills that are evidence based, skills that make it easier for clinicians to engage families effectively in the treatment process.

The underlying assumption of the approach described in this book is that for the majority of people, psychiatric symptoms or illnesses evolve in a social context. Understanding the social context of the presenting problem is critical to biopsychosocial formulation and treatment planning. Families can be helpful in identifying the history, precipitants, and likely future obstacles to the management of presenting problems. Families also play an important role, whether openly acknowledged or not, in the ongoing treatment process.

Patients typically will spend anywhere from 10 to 50 minutes every few weeks to every few months with their psychiatrists. In contrast, patients will be with their significant others for a much greater time. It seems shortsighted not to try to engage those people in the therapeutic process who can be helpful or hurtful, supportive or undermining of treatment outside the therapist's office.

Unique features of this book are 1) an organizing method that provides a unifying framework throughout the book, 2) clarification of the clinical decision-making process involved in establishing the level and extent of family involvement in patient care in different clinical settings, and 3) emphasis on an ongoing biopsychosocial formulation.

The overall approach is one that facilitates problem solving. The organizing framework applied with all families, regardless of the presenting problem(s) or the clinical setting in which the patient is seen, consists of the following six stages:

1. **Orientation:** Why are we here? What do we expect will happen?
2. **Assessment:** What are the problems from everybody's perspective?
3. **Biopsychosocial formulation:** Synthesis of the problems that is agreed to by the family and the therapist.
4. **Contracting:** What do you want to do about the identified problems? What has been stopping you?
5. **Treatment:** Work on agreed-upon tasks and assignments. Deal with obstacles and resistances to change.
6. **Closure:** What have we learned? Where do we go from here?

Current Psychiatric Practice

There is a significant need for a manual to guide psychiatrists in working with families of their patients. Psychiatrists are less and less likely to learn the art of family therapy. Psychiatrists who do want to work with families need a clear and readily understandable model for the assessment and treatment of families, one that is time limited and that can be adapted to different clinical settings and different patient populations. The family assessment and intervention model also needs to be compatible with biomedical and psychological treatments.

The currently predominant conceptual framework for the understanding of the etiology and treatment of psychiatric disorders is a biomedical one. The biomedical model emphasizes the role of neuroanatomical, neurophysiological, and neurochemical systems in the genesis and expression of mental illness and implies a pharmacological treatment approach. The role of psychological and social factors is acknowledged but thought to be of secondary importance. Because of the seemingly peripheral influence of psychosocial forces on psychiatric disorders, treatment with talking therapies is often referred to nonmedical mental health professionals. This trend is being reconsidered as it has become more evident that a narrow treatment focus (e.g., pharmacotherapy) by itself has limited effectiveness, that is, less effectiveness than combining drugs with psychotherapy.

Various trends have reinforced the biomedical model of psychiatric care. The medicalization of psychiatry and the limitation of the provision of psychosocial treatments by psychiatrists have been reinforced by insurance reimbursement systems. It is financially more advantageous, for instance, to provide three or four pharmacological management sessions per hour than to provide psychotherapy or family therapy in the same time frame.

The seductiveness of the biomedical model and its attendant focus on biological treatments are also reinforced by the relative ease of providing pharmacotherapy, for both psychiatrists and patients, as opposed to conducting psychosocial treatments. Psychiatrists can feel active and powerful by providing potent medicines. It is gratifying to be able to do something concrete, such as writing prescriptions, for patients. Providing medication management has been, up until recently, a unique function of psychiatrists, something that sets them apart from other mental health professionals. This exclusive prerogative has undergone some changes recently with the provision of licensing to prescribe medications by clinical nurse specialists and, in some states, by psychologists as well. Patients are seduced by the seeming ease with which they can resolve emotional distress merely by taking medications without having to work on changing ways of coping or relating to others. The expectation of the effectiveness of a "quick fix" with minimum effort is also syntonic with modern Western culture.

It is not surprising, then, that many established psychiatrists and those newly entering the profession do not consider it worthwhile to learn and practice psychosocial treatments. There has been a recent movement to make sure that newly trained psychiatrists have at least "core competence" in some forms of psychotherapy (1). Cognitive-behavioral therapy and interpersonal therapy training have received the most attention because these treatments have been presented in manual forms so as to be testable in treatment outcome studies. Such studies have supported the usefulness of these psychotherapies for a number of psychiatric disorders, either as monotherapy or in combination with pharmacotherapy. In reality, however, largely for economic reasons, most psychiatrists are likely to refer their patients who need psychotherapy to psychotherapists of various training as opposed to delivering those therapies themselves.

With increasing subspecialization in psychiatry (e.g., geriatric, forensic, consultation/liaison, substance abuse, psychopharmacology), we are in danger of losing track of the patient in his or her totality. That totality often involves the patient's significant others, people who are knowledgeable about the patient and the illness and who may be instrumental in supporting or obstructing the patient's treatment. Inattention to the family is likely to result in a skewed formulation of the patient's problems and thus a potentially limited treatment plan. Moreover, inadequate response to pharmacotherapy may be the result of a too-narrow case formulation; switching or augmenting medications will still not address personality issues or interpersonal problems. The current practice of polypharmacy may be partly a consequence of such a one-dimensional treatment approach.

The pharmaceutical industry, for understandable economic reasons, has strongly supported the medicalization of psychiatric care. Drug companies have done this through direct public advertising, through the domination of continuing medical education activities for physicians, through the funding of studies designed to showcase the importance of short-term and long-term pharmacological treatment using their products, and by supporting "thought leaders" in the field to disseminate information in a more acceptable way than can be achieved by advertising or by sales representatives alone. There is no such support for working with families.

Family-Oriented Patient Care

Family therapy skills are still not part of the "core competency" requirements for residency training programs. Many psychiatrists are uneasy about meeting with family members except for the gathering of historical information. Family interventions are delegated to social workers or family therapists. The reluctance of psychiatrists to participate in family interventions is surprising given extensive evidence supporting the significant role social environment plays in the onset and course of many psychiatric disorders. Why is there such reluctance by psychiatrists to engage in therapeutic work with families?

Part of the reason relates to the biomedical model and the socioeconomic forces outlined earlier. There are other reasons. Families can be perceived as being more threatening than individuals. To some extent, this is simply a function of the number of people in the room. The greater the number of people, the more difficult it may be to control them. To make the situation even more potentially threatening, many family members do not see themselves as patients and may assume a more equal and less deferential role with the therapist than an individual patient. Many family members also want explanations for what is or is not being done for their loved ones. Physicians are less used to, and may be uncomfortable with, having to explain their formulations and treatment plans to a potentially critical and demanding audience. A vicious circle can be readily established. In anticipation of an uncomfortable situation and without adequate training in family interventions, the psychiatrist avoids family members. The family members, wanting information and wanting to be involved in the care of their loved one, become critical. The psychiatrist avoids having to deal with such a demanding family. As a result, the patient's treatment may be compromised.

Early iterations of some family therapy models blamed families for illness in their loved ones. There may still be a residue of such thinking in some psychiatrists. Family members may also be hypersensitive to implications that they may contribute to the presenting illness, resulting in an increased likelihood of antagonistic interactions between families and psychiatrist.

Another historical residue inhibiting psychiatrists from meeting with families may be issues of transference in the therapeutic relationship and concerns about patient confidentiality. Some psychiatrists feel uneasy allowing outside persons to influence the therapeutic relationship. This may include family members. It is not uncommon to hear family members complain that they have not been allowed to participate in the care of their loved ones. Some psychiatrists also feel that talking to family members with or about the patient is a potential breach of confidentiality and are reluctant to do so even with the patient's permission. We believe that in most cases, this is countertherapeutic.

The research evidence for the effectiveness of family therapy in the treatment of psychiatric disorders is less extensive than the evidence for the effectiveness of individual psychotherapy. Family therapy is harder to put into manual form; few treatment manuals are readily available, and there are also fewer objective instruments to assess and measure family functioning than is the case for psychotherapy. This shortage of measures has limited the number of treatment outcome studies that could show the benefit of family interventions for various psychiatric disorders. The lack of outcome studies showing such benefit for family interventions has also contributed to the underutilization of family therapy by psychiatrists. This situation is in stark contrast to the period in the history of psychiatric treatment when claims for the effectiveness of family therapy were overstated—claims based on small sample sizes or case reports by a few charismatic psychiatrists, as was also the case for individual therapy. Controlled studies showing the effectiveness of family therapy are increasing in numbers.

Specific Family Assessment and Intervention Model

In this book we highlight evidence for including the family in the treatment of patients and provide suggestions for ways of doing so. The focus is on practical and evidence-based approaches. There are many different schools of family and couples therapy, just as there are many different schools of individual psychotherapy. We focus on what different family therapy models have in common rather than what sets them apart. We believe there are certain nonspecific common factors in the different schools of effective family therapies that are likely to be more important for treatment outcome than the specific maneuverings of a given form of therapy or of a particular family therapist. Some of the common goals of family therapies include the following:

- Increased knowledge
- Decreased guilt
- Redefinition of problems
- Increased use of adaptive coping mechanisms
- Appropriate emotional experience and communication
- Improvement of communication skills, problem-solving skills, and parenting skills
- Clarification of boundaries
- Setting of appropriate boundaries between familial subsystems and family of origin
- Insight regarding current transactions and historical factors
- Decreased conflict
- Work on family-of-origin issues (2)

There is nonetheless value in having one "umbrella" model that can help to frame family approaches to provide coherence, consistency, and conceptual ease. It is not possible for most therapists to learn to practice multiple family therapy models well unless they are doing family therapy most of the time.

They risk confusion, inconsistency, and getting lost in details. An overriding framework that allows for individual variation in technique and style can be reassuring to the therapist as well as to the family.

The model that we have chosen as our organizing principle is the McMaster Model of Family Functioning (3). We have chosen the McMaster Model for a variety of reasons. The McMaster Model has withstood the test of time. It has evolved over 40 years of research, practice, and teaching. It offers a comprehensive and integrated model of assessment and treatment that is teachable and testable. It provides a normative description of family functioning; it is multidimensional, focusing on many areas of family life; and it has validated instruments that can assess family functioning from an internal as well as an external perspective. The McMaster Model also has a treatment component, Problem-Centered Systems Therapy of the Family (PCSTF), that has been described in manual form and tested in treatment outcome studies. Other family therapy models will also be described and their active components outlined if they have been found to be useful.

We do not separate couples and family therapy into different treatment models. For us, the principles and clinical techniques for dealing with more than one person at a time in a treatment session are more similar than different to each other whether that involves two family members or more. We find it clinically helpful to see as many family members as are available and are interested in the care of their loved ones.

The core feature of the PCSTF used as the framework for assessing and treating families in this book is an emphasis on following defined and progressive stages in the process rather than focusing on specific techniques, etiologic theories, or unique personality styles of therapists. The major stages in working with families are Assessment, Contracting, Treatment, and Closure. These stages provide a progressive road map and a structure within which the therapist can be comprehensive without getting bogged down in peripheral details. One of the main challenges in meeting with families is to try to listen to many different perspectives while simultaneously keeping track of the various transactional patterns that are unfolding. A systematic structured conceptual framework is a great help in meeting that challenge.

The Assessment stage includes delineation of what family members identify as problems they are struggling with, the therapist's formulation of how these problems relate to the presenting problem of the identified patient, and the establishment of agreement between the therapist and all family members about this formulation. (**An example of the Assessment stage is shown in scene 3 and scenes 6–11 in the DVD.**)

The Contracting stage solicits the family's intent with regard to what they want to do about their problems, what has been stopping them from dealing with the problems effectively, and their commitment to agreed-upon steps to take in working toward a mutually acceptable resolution. (**For an example, see scene 14 in the DVD.**)

The Treatment stage occurs when the family works on the agreed-upon tasks and the therapist helps them to identify and overcome obstacles and resistances. (**For an example, see scene 14 in the DVD.**)

In the Closure stage there is a review and wrap-up of the therapy process and discussion of how to anticipate and deal with potential recurrences of the problems.

Not all stages need to be completed with all families. At minimum, most patients and their families should have an assessment. Some will move on to make changes based on the assessment, whereas others will need and want family treatment. Contracting and treatment, however, cannot take place without a proper assessment.

We show how families of patients with different psychiatric illnesses can be readily assessed and treated in different clinical settings and at different phases of their illness. We review different assessment tools, different formatting of family meetings, and ways of combining family approaches with pharmacotherapy and individual psychotherapy, Finally, we discuss ways of providing training in family interventions.

Conclusion

Despite the current emphasis on neurosciences, including functional MRIs, genomics, and targeted pharmaceutical agents, patients continue to experience their illness in a very personal way and within a social context. The effectiveness of medical treatments in psychiatry continues to be limited for many patients. Awareness of the limitations of the treatments and of the broader psychosocial context in which psychiatric illnesses are embedded is a call for including the families of patients in the treatment process.

Not all families need family therapy, and not all psychiatrists need to become family therapists. Talking to and meeting with the significant others of most patients, however, is a productive and ultimately time-saving exercise. In that meeting an assessment of the social system clarifies the context of the presenting problem and identifies strengths and supports that can make the treatment process more effective and less burdensome for the psychiatrist as well as the patient. An assessment, information-gathering, and information-sharing meeting may suffice for a large percentage of patients, especially those who have supportive and understanding families. The meeting is not likely to happen, however, if the psychiatrist is not comfortable meeting with families because he or she does not have a framework for evaluating families or the skills to do so. The goal of this book is to help make such meetings more likely to happen.

References

1.   Berman EM, Heru A, Grunebaum H, et al: Family skills for general psychiatry residents: meeting ACGME core competency requirements. Group for the Advancement of Psychiatry Committee on the Family. Acad Psychiatry 30:69–78, 2006

2.   Glick I, Berman E, Clarkin J, et al: Marital and Family Therapy, 4th Edition. Washington, DC, American Psychiatric Press, 2000

3.   Ryan CE, Epstein N, Keitner GI, et al: Evaluating and Treating Families: The McMaster Approach. New York, Routledge Taylor & Francis Group, 2005

2

Healthy Family Functioning

- Healthy family functioning is the ability to accomplish tasks that are important for the family's well-being, to adapt to changing circumstances, and to balance the needs of the individual and the family system.
- A family may have areas of healthy and unhealthy functioning.
- It is important to identify resilience and strengths in families.

To treat families effectively, therapists need to have some concept of what falls within the normal range of functioning and what types of behaviors and approaches should raise concern and indicate the need for intervention. Therapists need to know what constitutes healthy family functioning in order to understand deviations from it. Although the concept of normality may be self-evident, what constitutes "normal" in terms of family functioning is open to many perspectives.

It is difficult enough to describe a healthy or normal individual. When one is attempting to describe a healthy or normal family, the variables to consider multiply exponentially. Variables include the interaction between members of the family, the interaction of the family with the surrounding culture, the biology of the individuals concerned, and the expectation of the person doing the evaluating. Nevertheless, a working definition of what is generally acceptable is required in order to evaluate the need for some sort of intervention and the particular areas of family domains to be targeted by such intervention.

Concepts of health

- Absence of pathology
- Statistical average associated with good family function
- Ability to perform desired functions

A number of different definitions of normality have been advanced (1). Normality can be defined as the absence of pathology. If there are no symptoms or disorder in any family member, then the family can be thought of as functioning in a healthy way. However, just as the prevalence of symptoms may not necessarily imply family pathology, lack of symptoms in family members may not necessarily imply healthy family functioning. There are situations in which families accept certain behavioral patterns without evidence of distress or dysfunction, that may nonetheless be of potential risk to them. Examples of this can be seen in families where risky behaviors (such as substance abuse) or safety issues (such as clear expectations about driving and/or the presence of dangerous materials in the home) are left undefined.

Normality may also be defined in terms of a statistical average. Measurements are made on a particular sample and the average score is taken to represent the normal score for that population. If the sample is representative of the total population, then something is known of the distribution of the characteristic being measured across the population as a whole. However, frequency distributions of certain family functions such as discussing financial problems does not tell us much that is useful about any individual family. Furthermore, family functions that are common may not be healthy.

One useful perspective on normality is to think of those functions that are healthy or ideal in terms of accomplishing important family functions. A healthy family is able to accomplish important family functions, which lead to the successful development and well-being of family members. A well-functioning family meets the diverse needs of its members but also adapts these needs to the individual characteristics of the various members. In other words, there is a fit between the way families are able to accomplish their goals and a particular style or temperament of the individual family members. It is the fit between the needs of the individual and the system as a whole that makes them successful.

Family Functions

The primary function of a family is to provide a safe setting for the development and maintenance of family members' social, psychological, and biological needs (2). In the course of fulfilling these functions, families have to deal with a variety of issues, problems, or tasks, which can be grouped as follows: basic task areas, developmental task areas, and hazardous task areas.

Basic task areas include the provision of food, money, transportation, and shelter by the family members for each other. *Developmental task areas* encompass the growth of individuals within a family over a period of time and the capacity of the family system to encourage and nourish such growth. Stages of growth include the challenges of infancy, childhood, adolescence, middle age, and old age. On a family level, developmental tasks can include stages such as the beginning of marriage, bringing up young children, dealing with job changes, the last child leaving home, retirement issues, and handling aging. *Hazardous tasks areas* involve family crises arising from illness, accident, and loss of income, job change, and other threats to the integrity of the family. Families that are unable to deal effectively with these tasks areas are most likely to develop clinically significant problems and chronic maladapted family functioning.

Historical Trends

The structure and function of the family change with and adapt to the economic, social, and cultural forces of the times. The role of parents, children, and the extended family has and will continue to vary and needs to be taken into consideration when assessing the capacity of a family to deal with and adapt to the demands made on it not only by the individual needs of the family members but also by society at large.

At different times in history, men and women have played different roles within the family in terms of their responsibilities in and out of the home and also in terms of expectations of their intimacy with each other. Similarly, expectations of the roles and functions of children have varied from being contributors to the family's economic health to being dependent on the family for long periods. Extended family members have at some times been great sources of mutual support and at other times unavailable because of their own commitments or geographical distance due to increasing mobility.

A smaller family generally characterizes the current sociocultural family paradigm in Western society, with parents spending more time together before and after the birth of children. This trend, along with decreased availability of extended family members, has led to increased expectations for emotional connectedness between partners. Women's roles have changed dramatically, most would agree for the better for them and for their families. A large percentage of women are in the workforce outside the home and are redefining their expectations from society as well as from their spouses to include greater autonomy and authority. At the same time, increased pressure to function as caretakers at home and as productive employees/employers creates new stresses and needs for support. Men are expected to be more involved in the practical and emotional life of the family. With fewer children, each child becomes more valued and shifts from being an economic advantage to an economic burden for the family. Increasing longevity creates new challenges in forcing people to learn how to meet each other's needs over prolonged time periods and through many phases in their family life cycle. The near normalization of divorce has created new opportunities as well as risks for couples as they weigh their options in dealing with family pressures.

Family functions

- Problem solving
- Communication
- Role allocation
- Affective responsiveness
- Affective involvement
- Behavior control

There are effective ways of dealing with these changing social and interpersonal forces. Healthy families have found approaches in problem solving that allow them to react to and shape their external and internal environments so as to feel satisfied that their individual and family needs are being reasonably met. Unhealthy families have trouble finding a balance that accommodates to their personal needs while maintaining the integrity of the family system. The difference lies not only in the solution but also in the process of solving the problem.

Dimensions of Family Functioning

Healthy family functioning should be defined proactively in terms of positive successful family interactional patterns. It is helpful to think of constructive ways of dealing with the world by subdividing family function into specific areas that represent the family's way of addressing the aforementioned task areas that all families face. Six family dimensions have been described that provide a reasonably comprehensive view of the ways in which families deal with each other and the world around them (3). These dimensions include problem solving, communication, role allocation, affective responsiveness, affective involvement, and behavior control. **Part One in the accompanying DVD (scenes 6–11) shows how each of these dimensions is assessed in a family with a member who has depressive symptoms.** No single dimension predicts good or poor family functioning, but for each of these dimensions one can postulate more or less effective ways of dealing with the challenges of family life.

In evaluating families it is important to look for strengths and effectiveness as well as for dysfunction. It is much easier to bring about clinical change by reinforcing already available functional transactional patterns than by trying to create new ways of dealing with each other or by criticizing existing deficiencies.

Problem Solving

Problem solving refers to a family's ability to resolve problems to a level that maintains effective family functioning. Family problems can be divided into *instrumental* problems and *affective* problems. Instrumental problems relate to issues that are basic in nature such as the provision of money, food, clothing, housing, and transportation. Affective problems relate to issues of emotional feeling such as anger or depression that may arise in families. Families whose functioning is disrupted by instrumental problems rarely deal effectively with affective problems. Families whose functioning is disrupted by affective problems, however, may still deal adequately with instrumental problems. Effective families solve most problems efficiently and relatively easily. These families can readily identify problems. They can communicate with appropriate people about the problem and possible alternative solutions. They are able to choose alternatives and carry out the actions required by that choice. They tend to monitor the outcome to ensure that it was successful and evaluate its effectiveness when the problem is resolved.

Well-functioning families can still have minor unresolved problems. Such minor problems, however, do not create ongoing disruptions within the family. Families can also progress through various stages of problem solving at a different pace and still maintain a high level of functioning as long as they eventually are able to resolve the presenting problems. The best-functioning families are able to deal with both instrumental and affective problems comparably well, whereas less well functioning families can deal with instrumental problems well but have more trouble with affective problems. Families that cannot even deal well with instrumental problems are the least well functioning and are barely able to deal with the affective issues that percolate through their family.

Communication

Effective communication is a central issue in family functioning models. Communication is defined as the exchange of information within a family. Communication can also be divided into instrumental and affective areas and can be described as clear or masked and direct or indirect. The clear versus masked continuum focuses on whether the content of the message is clearly stated or camouflaged, muddy, or vague. The direct versus indirect continuum focuses on whether messages go through the appropriate individuals or tend to be deflected to other people.

Healthy families tend to communicate in a clear and direct manner in both instrumental and affective areas. There can be brief occasions of hesitation or beating around the bush (this is called *masking*). Family members may on occasion not clearly state a personal point of view (this is called *indirect communication*). However, in well-functioning families, family members feel free to discuss issues with each other, are respectful of differences of opinion, address each other directly, and express their feelings to each other without fear of retribution or misunderstanding.

Role Allocation

Family roles are defined as repetitive patterns of behavior by which family members fulfill family functions. There are broad ranges of family functions that need to be addressed. These include the provision of resources such as food, clothing, and shelter. Families also need to provide nurturing and support for each other in the form of comfort, warmth, and reassurance. Adults in families need to be able to gratify each other sexually. Families need to ensure the possibility of personal development via each family member's social development as well as peer development.

The family system also needs ongoing maintenance in management. Leadership within a family needs to be defined and struggles over leadership resolved. Families need to define boundaries relating to extended family, friends, neighbors, external institutions, and agencies. Rules regarding what is or is not acceptable within the family by the various family members need to be established and enforced. Household finances need to be regulated and sustained. The physical health of individuals within the family need to be ensured by setting up and keeping medical appointments, identifying health problems, and maintaining compliance with treatment regimens.

Role allocation and accountability also need to be considered. Role allocation is defined as the family's patterns of assigning roles to various family members. Families have to ensure that roles and tasks are assigned to those who are able to fulfill them. Assignments should be done clearly and explicitly and should be changeable as circumstances dictate. Roles should also be distributed in a way that is acceptable and seen as fair by all family members. Role accountability involves the procedures in the family for making sure that functions are fulfilled.

Well-functioning families ensure that all necessary family functions are fulfilled. Allocation of responsibilities within the family is reasonable and does not overburden one or more members. Accountability for following through on assigned responsibilities is made clear. There are clear avenues whereby families can renegotiate various role functions that have been assigned to them and family members not feel unduly overburdened by tasks and responsibilities relative to other family members.

As with other family domains, family functions can span a range of effectiveness that is not necessarily optimal. What makes them still effective, however, is that they do not lead to persistent conflict. Most functions in the family can be shared, although certain individuals may carry what seems to be a disproportionate load as long as they do not feel taken advantage of by that process. Imbalances in role functions in the family can be offset by compensation in other areas of family life and/or by redistribution of loads over time as the imbalance becomes apparent.

Affective Responsiveness

Affective responsiveness assesses whether individual family members can demonstrate an ability to respond with the full spectrum of feelings experienced by human beings. It also considers whether the emotion experienced is consistent with the stimulus provided or the situational context in which it emerges. Two categories of affect can be evaluated: *welfare emotions* consist of affection, warmth, tenderness, support, love, consolation, happiness, and joy, whereas *emergency emotions* consist of anger, fear, sadness, disappointment, and depression.

In healthy families individuals possess the capacity to experience and express a full range of emotions. Emotional expression is of reasonable intensity and duration so as not to cause persistent anxiety and avoidance in other family members. Although there may be individual family members who have more or less capacity to experience a particular affect, well-functioning families are able to accommodate to this in a way that does not disrupt their own functioning. It is important to recognize that certain individuals are more or less able to experience and express different kinds of affect. The recognition of the capabilities and limitations of individual family members and the ability to accommodate to that reality are part of what defines a well-functioning family.

Affective Involvement

Affective involvement describes the extent to which family members show interest in and value the particular activities and interests of other family members. Styles can range from a total lack of involvement at one end of the continuum to extreme involvement at the other. In well-functioning families there is empathic involvement with other family members. There is interest in the other for the sake of the other, not for what one can get out of it for oneself. Even in healthy families there may be individuals who are more self-absorbed and less sensitive to the needs of others. But in well-functioning families, other family members are able to adapt and adjust in a way that does not allow persistent conflicts to manifest themselves in that family.

Behavior Control

Behavior control is the pattern that a family adopts for handling behavior in three areas: physically dangerous situations, situations that involve meeting and expressing psychobiological needs and drives, and situations involving interpersonal socializing behavior between both family members and people outside the family. This dimension reflects the standards or rules that the family sets in these areas and the latitude allowed individuals within a family relative to these standards. Families can be rigid, flexible, laissez-faire, or chaotic. Well-functioning families tend to use flexible means of dealing with behavioral expectations within the family. These families tend to be clear about the rules within the family but allow for negotiation and adjustment of the rules while maintaining consistency over time. Disagreements between family members can occur, but they have ways of resolving them. Well-functioning families do not try to suppress the rules by soliciting different perspectives from various family members.

Having a normative view of the various dimensions of family functioning can help a therapist understand to what extent the family they are dealing with matches such expectations. There are clear cultural assumptions embedded in the formulations outlined above, but the principles can be applied to different cultural situations. The key issue may not be what a particular culture expects from the family but to what extent a family within a given culture is able to negotiate what they expect from each other and from the culture outside the family.

Marital and Family Life Cycle

The demands on family systems vary over the family's life cycle, depending on its stage of development (4). The family faces different demands at different points of time; however, families that are well functioning in the areas outlined above are able to meet these demands because of intrinsic structures and ways of dealing with systems that they have been able to evolve in an effective manner. Other families that have less effective coping skills in some of the dimensions outlined are more likely to have difficulties negotiating their way through the various stages of family life. Well-functioning families' members feel connected and committed to each other. They are mutually supportive. Individuals respect each other's differences and foster each other's autonomy and separate needs, even within the context of the family system. Well-functioning families support effective parental leadership to ensure the provision of nurturance and protection, particularly by caring for children and other vulnerable family members. Well-functioning families have organizational stability characterized by clarity, consistency, and predictability. Such families are adaptable, flexibly meeting internal and external demands for change. They tend to communicate openly with each other and have clear rules and expectations. They have a full range of emotional expressiveness and empathic connections. Well-functioning families have effective problem-solving and conflict resolution processes. Families function better when they have economic security and support from extended kin and friendship networks as well as from the community at large. Also, a shared belief system connects families to past and future generations' ethical values, along with concern for the larger human community, and helps to enhance healthy family functioning.

In the following sections we outline healthy family functioning for a "modal" family, recognizing that there are many variations. There are a number of other specific types of family situations cutting across the life cycle (divorce, gay couples, blended families) that present their own set of challenges and opportunities. These are discussed in Chapter 12.

Individual Life Cycle

Family issues are strongly affected by the age of adult members. Their particular developmental stage and the life issues that they are dealing with by necessity affect the family system. Having knowledge of the areas of concern at different stages of the life cycle can help the therapist understand and put into better context problems they are likely to encounter in families.

Adult developmental phases can be divided roughly into early adulthood (age 20–40 years), mid-adulthood (age 40–60 years), and older adulthood (age 60 years and older). Table 2–1 presents components of adult development and the family life cycle.

Early Adulthood

The tasks of early adulthood include launching from one's family of origin and developing a sense of identity, life structure, career track, and movement toward an intimate and committed relationship. Relationships with parents are renegotiated. By age 30–40 years, there is a tendency to settle into a chosen life structure with a deepened commitment to work and intimate relationships. With the birth of children, the pleasures and pressures of taking care of the family, in addition to advancing in the workplace, create the need for being able to handle multiple responsibilities. Pressures to fulfill role expectations in these multiple domains while finding enough time for individual pursuits become more complicated. Successful transition in these phases allows individuals to experience themselves as fully adult.

Mid-Adulthood

In this stage individuals become more comfortable with their multiple roles and if successful have a greater sense of effectiveness and competence. For some, there may be a need to reevaluate work goals and relationships, leading at times to some midlife transitions and anxiety surrounding this reevaluation. There is a tendency over time to accept what one has become and to begin to deal with the reality of aging and mortality. It is also a time when individuals may need to take care not only of their children but also of their parents.

Older Adulthood

In this stage individuals begin to review their lives more systematically. They may gradually transition from feeling a need to be in charge to providing more support for the next generation. Medical problems and the reality of physical limitations as a result of aging need new accommodations. With the

Table 2–1.   The family life cycle and adult development

Early adulthood (age 20–40 years)	Mid-adulthood (age 40–60 years)	Older adulthood (age 60+ years)
Age 20–30 years 1. Establish an independent life structure—home, friends, etc. 2. Renegotiate relationships with parents 3. Make first set of decisions around occupational choice 4. Explore intimacy/sexuality 5. Possibly deal with parenthood **Age 30 transition** Sometimes rethink early choices—"course correction" **Age 30–40 years** 1. Settle into chosen life structure 2. Deepen commitment to work and intimate relationships 3. Experience self as fully adult	**Age 40–50 years** 1. Deal with complexities of being command generation: may be responsible for children and/or aging parents 2. Midlife transition: reevaluate life goals, work, and relationships 3. Forgive self for sins of omission and commission **Age 50–60 years** 1. Settle into life one chose in 40s 2. Accept who one has become 3. Deal with grandparenthood 4. Deal with issues of aging and mortality	**Age 60+ years** 1. Conduct a life review 2. Give up being command generation 3. Find function and direction in a world that values youth 4. Deal with physical changes of aging **Age 75+ years** Focus on functioning despite physical aging

Source.   Reprinted from Glick ID, Berman EM, Clarkin JF, et al: "Understanding the Functional Family," in *Marital and Family Therapy,* 4th Edition. Washington, DC, American Psychiatric Press, 2000, p 63. Used with permission.

possibility of retirement, finding new meaning in life becomes important. This can lead to philosophical and spiritual development.

Family Life Cycle

Marriages and families also go through various stages of evolution and development, each of which presents its own unique challenges and satisfactions. It is helpful to have some conception of these different phases to better understand the issues that a particular family may be presenting.

Courtship and Early Marriage

Couple formation is best done when both individuals have completed the tasks of restructuring their relationship with their parents, learned enough about themselves to become aware of their characteristic problems, and had enough freedom and adventure that the demands of an intense relationship feel comforting rather than constrictive. They must establish an identity as a couple, develop effective ways of communicating and solving problems, and begin to establish a mutual pattern of relating to parents, friends, and work. Competency at intimate life, work life, and parenting needs to develop simultaneously. In general, marital satisfaction is greatest in the first years and begins to decline, reaching a low point when the children become adolescents. However, divorces are also highest in the first year as the marriages of poorly matched couples dissolve. Common stress points in early adult marriages are child bearing, attempting an egalitarian marriage in a nonegalitarian culture, and enduring midlife transitions as one or both partners go through a period of reevaluating themselves.

Individuals often enter into a marriage with unrealistic expectations. Individuals tend to want somebody who is familiar and comfortable—in other words, like themselves—while at the same time hoping that the other person will complement and complete those parts of themselves that they feel are deficient or problematic. A lack of acceptance of individual differences between couples leads to attempts by one individual to make the other more like them, often resulting in conflict and disappointment.

Lewis (5) has described five dimensions important in determining the quality of a marital relationship. These include, first, the question of power and who is in charge. Second, partners need to establish the degree of closeness or distance and the amount of shared activities and values that they are comfortable with. Third, boundaries need to be applied to determine who is included or excluded from the marital/family system. Fourth, partners need to feel equally committed to their relationship and to the family unit. Fifth, partners also need to negotiate the degree of intimacy that they are comfortable with and the degree to which they are willing to share their respective vulnerabilities.

Children

With the arrival of children, families tend to become closer, with an intense inward focus on the children. Roles need to be redefined. Family boundaries need to be loosened to allow extended family members to participate in the enjoyment of and the sharing of responsibilities of caring for the children. It can be difficult for parents to find sufficient time for each other with multiple demands of work, home maintenance, and parenting.

As children become adolescents, they press for greater autonomy. Parents also begin to struggle with contradictory desires for family closeness and safety on the one hand and freedom on the other. Families at this stage must be strong, flexible, and able to support growth. They need to be able to maintain boundaries and limits while at the same time allowing their children increasing exploration and autonomy. For the majority of well-functioning families, however, adolescence is not a time of chaos and rebellion.

The family needs to evolve as adolescents turn into young adults. Families need to continue the letting-go process by restructuring relationships to allow for more autonomy while continuing to be related and connected in a meaningful way.

In healthy families the basic roles and functions necessary for family adaptation are carried out by their subsystems (e.g., marital, spousal, sibling). These subsystems can be categorized according to the division of labor, or psychosocial tasks within the family. For example, spouses generally offer each other social and emotional companionship and sexual intimacy, whereas parents provide nurturance, support, and guidance for children. In the sibling subsystem, children learn to share, trust, negotiate for resources, and develop social skills. Children provide parents with loyalty and a sense of purpose. The family subsystems are arranged not only functionally but also hierarchically, with parents typically occupying positions of authority in relation to their offspring.

Empty Nest

As children leave home, parents need to be able to redefine their roles and priorities. It is an opportunity for parents to spend more time together, to feel less pressured, and to explore individual interests. It is also a time of potential distress when interpersonal problems between the parents that had been sidelined by focusing on the needs of the children may surface. There is a need at this life stage to redefine goals and meaning while at the same time finding ways of connecting more closely to one's partner. **Scene 4 in the DVD shows how illness in one family member can influence the decision of an adult child to return home.**

Retirement

Another significant period of role transition in the family is when one or both partners in a relationship retire. This is a life stage that promises both new opportunities and challenges. Retirement requires individuals to redefine their identity and place in society. The solution to these challenges inevitably affects relationships. Finding new interests and goals and feeling connected and useful allow for successful enjoyment of new leisure time. Couples have to find ways of managing the increased amount of time they spend together. They have to find ways of being together that are supportive without being enmeshed or too confining. The health and financial stability of the couple will have a major impact on their ability to experience this stage of their lives in a satisfying way.

Death and Grieving

As couples age and health problems increase, they will increasingly have to deal with the death of friends, their partner, and eventually themselves. There are many challenges at this stage of life. Individuals have to come to terms with their own mortality and find ways of resolving issues of importance to them before dying. They are likely to be worried about the health of their partner and experience fears of loss, dependence, and isolation. Couples need to find ways of discussing their concerns and plan together how they want to deal with the problems they are likely to face. The involvement of children and extended family members can ease many concerns. Unfortunately, unresolved family problems can make this process even more difficult.

Family Resilience

Aspects of family resilience

- Clear family organization
- Direct communication
- Cohesion, connectedness, and mutual support
- Positive adaptation to adversity

A family will inevitably have its strengths and weaknesses. Family strengths can protect against illnesses, and family weaknesses can predispose families to illnesses. For example, in a prospective, community-based study of 194 patients, having emotional support was associated with a better outcome among elderly patients hospitalized for acute myocardial infarction (6). Lack of emotional support was significantly associated with 6-month mortality (odds ratio = 2.9; 95% confidence interval 1.2 to 6.9), even after controlling for severity of myocardial infarction, comorbidity, sociodemographic factors, and risk factors such as smoking and hypertension.

Family strengths can also offset family difficulties. Parenting quality is a predictor for competency in children and adolescents. Academic achievement, conduct, and peer social competence were evaluated in 205 children who were followed for 10 years. Parenting quality was protective even in the context of severe adversity. Structure, rules, closeness, warmth, and high expectations for the child's achievement and prosocial behavior were the parenting qualities associated with higher levels of competency (7).

Families, however, are more complex than the presence or absence of certain positive or negative characteristics. A family's response to adversity can reveal internal resources that help the family emerge strengthened when faced with a stressor, such as family illness. Researchers have studied family processes to try to understand what goes on within families that enable them to cope well with adversity.

Family resilience is the interplay of multiple risk and protective factors that occur over time and involves individual, family, and other sociocultural influences (8). Initially, resilience research focused on individuals and followed them over the course of their lifetime. For example, 700 children of plantation workers living in poverty in Hawaii were followed into adulthood (9). By age 18, two-thirds of the children had done poorly but one-third had developed into competent, caring, and confident young adults. Through midlife, all but two of these competent adults were living successful lives. All the competent adults had a significant relationship with family members, partners, coaches, or teachers. These significant "family" relationships were thought to act as mediating protective factors that influenced the trajectory of these children's lives in positive ways. The positive family factors were found to influence individual resilience.

Family resilience implies that a family has an internal organization or has reorganized specifically to protect against stress. Many families report that through weathering a crisis together their relationships were enriched and became more loving than they might otherwise have been (10). In one study of families coping with a relative who had mental illness, 87.7% of families reported family resilience and 99.2% of family members reported personal resilience (11). One family member stated, "When a family experiences something like this, it makes for very compassionate people—people of substance. My brother created a bond among us that we will not allow to be broken."

Family resilience describes dynamic processes that foster positive adaptation to adversity. What is known about resilient families? High-functioning families have strong affiliative value (12) and approach adversity as a shared challenge. Cohesion or connectedness provides mutual support and collaboration among members when a family is facing a crisis (12, 13). Clear and direct communication facilitates effective functioning, which in turn facilitates good problem solving, an essential skill in times of adversity (3, 14). The key family processes thought to contribute to family resilience occur in three main domains: family belief systems, organizational patterns, and communication/problem solving (1).

In general medicine, family processes that influence chronic medical illness are outlined in a review commissioned by the Institute of Medicine and the National Academy of Sciences (15). Family protective processes linked to improved outcomes are family closeness, mutuality, connectedness, caregiver coping skills, mutually supportive family relationships, clear family organization, and direct communication about the illness and its management. Family factors and processes linked to poorer outcomes are interfamilial conflict, criticism and blame, perfectionism and rigidity, delayed family developmental tasks, lack of an extrafamilial support system, and psychological trauma related to diagnosis and treatment.

Family resilience is not immediately apparent; thus, assessing a family for the presence of family strengths or protective family processes is needed. In a study of caregivers attending a memory disorder clinic, many caregivers reported a sense of reward in caring for their relatives. These caregivers continued to report more reward than burden, even in the presence of deteriorating patient functioning (16). The caregivers reported "feeling needed and responsible," "feeling good inside," "doing for someone what you want for yourself," "knowing I've done my best," and "being able to help."

By focusing on family strengths and family resilience, the medical professional can engage families positively. Each physician can involve the family in the assessment process and can include family members in treatment planning. Many successful family interventions are educational, are applicable to all health care settings, and approach family members openly and collaboratively. Nationally, the promotion of health can be furthered by promoting good family functioning in the same way that diet, exercise, and healthy life habits are promoted for their preventative effects on health.

Conclusion

Each family should be approached as a unique cultural system that is influenced by ethnicity, race, religion, social class, and the immediate social context. To develop a clinically meaningful picture of family functioning, the therapist should evaluate the families along the dimensions we have outlined in this chapter. The goal of this assessment is to develop a formulation about the strengths of the family and areas that are perceived to be problematic by the family members and by the therapist in the course of his or her evaluation (Chapter 4). This formulation of the family's general functioning is the foundation for understanding the family's capacity to deal with the stresses that may be bringing them to professional attention. Understanding the range of functional and, in contrast, dysfunctional family interactional styles provides a context for the therapist and the family to develop agreed-upon goals for family interventions (Chapter 9).

References

1. Walsh F: Family resilience: a framework for clinical practice. Fam Process 42:1–18, 2003
2. Epstein NB, Levin S, Bishop DS: The family as a social unit. Can Fam Physician 22:1411–1413, 1976
3. Epstein N, Ryan CE, Bishop D, et al: The McMaster Model: a view of healthy family functioning, in Normal Family Processes: Growing Diversity and Complexity, 3rd Edition. Edited by Walsh F. New York, Guilford, 2003, pp 581–607
4. Glick I, Berman E, Clarkin J, et al: Marital and Family Therapy, 4th Edition. Washington, DC, American Psychiatric Press, 2000
5. Lewis JM: For better or worse: interpersonal relationship and individual outcome. Am J Psychiatry 155:582–589, 1998
6. Berkman L, Leo-Summers L, Horowitz RI: Emotional support and survival after myocardial infarction. Ann Intern Med 117:1003–1009, 1992
7. Masten AS, Hubbard JJ, Gest SD, et al: Competence in the context of adversity: pathways to resilience and maladaptation from childhood to late adolescence. Dev Psychopathol 11:143–169, 1999
8. Garmezy N: Resilience and vulnerability to adverse developmental outcomes associated with poverty. Am Behav Sci 34:416–430, 1991
9. Werner EE: Risk, resilience and recovery: perspectives from the Kauai study. Dev Psychopathol 5:503–515, 1993
10. Stinnett N, DeFrain J, DeFrain N: Good Families. New York, Doubleday, 1997
11. Marsh DT, Lefley HP: The family experience of mental illness: evidence for resilience. Psychiatr Rehabil J 20:3–12, 1996
12. Beavers R, Hampson RB: Successful Families: Assessment and Intervention. New York, WW Norton, 1990
13. Antonovsky A: Unraveling the Mystery of Health. San Francisco, CA, Jossey-Bass, 1987
14. Ryan CE, Epstein N, Keitner GI, et al: Evaluating and Treating Families: The McMaster Approach. New York, Routledge Taylor & Francis Group, 2005
15. Weihs K, Fisher L, Baird MA: Families, health and behavior. Fam Syst Health 20:7–46, 2002
16. Heru AM, Ryan CE, Iqbal A: Family functioning in the caregivers of patients with dementia. Int J Geriatr Psychiatry 19:533–537, 2004

3

Family Research

- Family and relational factors interact with biological systems to produce disease.
- The quality of relationships is known to influence the outcome of medical and psychiatric illnesses.
- Family intervention can be implemented successfully at all phases of illness: to prevent disease, to reduce chronicity, and to improve functioning in the chronic phase.
- The American Psychiatric Association Practice Guidelines delineate the benefits of family involvement in the acute and maintenance treatment of several illnesses, for example, schizophrenia, mood disorders, anxiety disorders, eating disorders, and substance abuse disorders.

This chapter outlines the family research that provides the rationale for assessing and treating family factors in medical and psychiatric illnesses. Family research is described under the following headings: relational factors and biological systems, relational factors and medical illnesses, and relational factors and psychiatric illnesses.

The evidence-based family interventions for both medical and psychiatric illnesses are reviewed under headings that reflect major areas of research: family intervention and the promotion of healthy behaviors and the prevention of illness; family interventions in the acute phase with the purpose of reducing chronicity; and family interventions and management of chronic illnesses.

It is only in the past decade that family research has established family psychiatry on a firm basis. Generally speaking, family researchers examine

31

specific family factors that are important in the etiology and maintenance of medical and psychiatric illnesses and evaluate evidence-based family treatments. These treatments can be either singular family therapies or integrated treatments that include a family component.

Families can be involved in the assessment and treatment of the patient at all stages of care. Families can be involved at varying depths, ranging from participating in psychoeducational programs to family treatment that involves change in relational functioning. Family research clearly demonstrates that working with the families of patients is an empirically valid practice.

Relational Factors and Biological Systems

The links between relational factors and specific biological processes that underlie disease processes are being clarified. For example, poor marital quality is associated with negative physical health outcomes through several mechanisms. First, social and health behaviors such as eating patterns and exercise habits influence health outcome. These patterns are often derived from family traditions and require the family to work together if changes are to occur. Second, early childhood family environment influences the expression of genetic vulnerability. The classic research in this area is described in the next section. Third, the cardiovascular, endocrine, and immune systems are influenced by psychological factors including the quality of family relationships.

Links between relational factors and biological processes

- Supportive environment modulates genetic expression.
- Social support reduces physiological reactivity to stress.
- Oxytocin reduces social stress.
- Good marriages are associated with better cardiovascular profiles.
- Caregivers experience premature aging of the immune system.

Relational Factors and Genetic Expression

Relational factors influence disease at the level of gene expression. Specific relational/familial patterns protect or place a person at risk for the development of an illness to which the person is genetically vulnerable. Studies of schizophrenia, conduct disorder, and depression have elucidated these factors.

The relational factors associated with increased risk for schizophrenia are high levels of family conflict, restricted affect, and poor definition of individual responsibilities and parental leadership (1). The presence of an adverse, adoptive rearing environment results in conduct disorder in children at biological risk (2). Biological risk is identified by severe antisocial personality disorder or alcoholism in the birth parents. Women developed depression only when the biological risk factor was combined with an adverse rearing environment (3). Women reared in an adverse environment such as severe parental psychopathology, marital difficulties, and legal problems developed depression more often than did women with biological risk but no adversity in childhood.

Relational Factors and the Cardiovascular System

Emotional support improves the outcome of patients with cardiac disease (4). In a study of hospitalized elderly patients with acute myocardial infarction, cardiac status was improved at 6-month follow-up if the patients had good emotional support (5). Good marital support also improved survival in 189 patients with heart failure, independent of illness severity. In this study, improved survival continued during an 8-year follow-up period ($P<0.001$), especially for female patients. Good marital support was a substantially better outcome indicator than individual risk and protective factors, such as psychological distress, hostility, neuroticism, self-efficacy, optimism, and breadth of perceived emotional support (6).

Marriage itself is well known to confer better health outcome for men, and recent evidence from a prospective study of 493 women from the Healthy Women Study has shown the same benefits for women. Women with high marital quality had improved cardiovascular risk profiles and illness trajectories with lower levels of biological, lifestyle, and psychosocial risk factors when compared with women who had moderate or low marital satisfaction or women who were single, divorced, and widowed (7). In contrast, marital conflict is associated with increased blood pressure and heart rate, thus increasing risk of cardiac disease (8).

Relational Factors and the Endocrine System

The hypothalamic-pituitary-adrenal (HPA) axis is a complex set of direct influences and feedback interactions that controls reactions to stress and regulates many body processes, including the immune system and emotions. The family environment and parental relational factors have been shown to act as a childhood stress and contribute to childhood illness. This has been most clearly shown in a study of 264 infants, children, adolescents, and young adults, ages 2 months to 18 years, residing in a rural Caribbean village. Biological, psychological, and health outcome data were measured over 9 years. Household income, land ownership, parental education, and other socioeconomic measures were weakly associated with childhood illness, and there was no evidence that higher socioeconomic status (improved housing, diet, workloads, and access to private health care) had direct effects on child health. However, unstable mating relationships of parents/caretakers and household composition were associated with abnormal glucocorticoid response profiles, diminished immunity, and frequent illness (9).

Physiological reactivity to stressors is influenced by social support. Study volunteers completed three tasks in which daily social support, neurocognitive reactivity to a social stressor, and neuroendocrine responses to a social stressor were assessed. Participants with social support showed diminished cortisol reactivity, reduced neurocognitive reactivity to social stressors, and reduced neuroendocrine stress responses (10).

Oxytocin modulates the stress response in both animals and humans. Oxytocin is released peripherally and within the brain in response to both physical and psychosocial stress; it also exerts inhibitory effects on the stress-induced activity of the HPA axis. During lactation, the suckling stimulus by the newborn increases oxytocin and induces a neuroendocrine hyporesponsiveness to physical and psychological situations that induce anxiety and stress, including attenuated secretion of adrenocorticotropic hormone, corticosterone, and catecholamine. In rhesus monkeys, disturbances in primary relationships change neural systems that control emotional resilience (11, 12). In rats, variations in maternal care affect the expression of oxytocin receptors, resulting in familial transmission of patterns of either high- or low-nurturing maternal behavior. The adult females with high levels of maternal licking and grooming as pups had increased oxytocin receptors in the central nucleus of the amygdala and bed nucleus of the stria terminalis (13).

Human experiments confirm the role of oxytocin in promoting positive social interactions. Oxytocin administered intranasally to healthy men enhanced the buffering effect of social support on stress responsiveness (14). In this study, men received oxytocin 50 minutes before a stressor and their responses were compared with those of men who received a placebo and no social support. Social support suppressed free cortical levels. Oxytocin produced an anxiolytic effect. The combination of oxytocin and social support produced the lowest cortisol concentrations as well as increased calmness and decreased anxiety during stress. These results posit a biological mechanism for the stress-protective effects of positive social interactions.

Clinical studies that examine how biological and psychosocial factors interact together are rare. However, one study exemplifies this approach to psychiatric illness. In this study of postpartum depression, progesterone levels and social support were evaluated in 160 women in the perinatal period (15). Progesterone concentrations had no direct effect on depressive symptoms but had indirect effects mediated through psychosocial stressors and symptoms of anxiety. The variance in depressive symptoms was accounted for by the indirect effects of biological risk factors on psychosocial variables and anxiety. In line with other research findings (see section on relational factors and genetic expression), it is hypothesized that biological variables alter a person's sensitivity to environmental stressors, such as lack of social support, and thus determine the threshold for developing symptoms. The lack of a direct relationship between progesterone concentrations and symptoms of depression during pregnancy explains the previous difficulties in identifying a linear relationship between hormonal variables and depression during the perinatal period. These relationships may only be apparent in the presence of relevant psychosocial stressors.

Relational Factors and the Immune System

Chronic stress, such as marital conflict, alters the sensitivity of the immune system and increases interleukin-6 production (16). Many conditions associated with aging, including cardiovascular disease, osteoporosis, arthritis, type 2 diabetes mellitus, certain lymphoproliferative diseases or cancers, Alzheimer's disease, and periodontal disease are associated with increased interleukin-6 production. Persistent stimulation of proinflammatory cytokine production has the greatest effect among older adults who already show age-related increases in interleukin-6 production. Increases in proinflammatory cytokines are associated with depressive disorders and anxiety, suggesting a mechanism linking depressive and anxiety symptoms to general health problems (17).

Children who live with parents who have psychiatric symptoms have more total illnesses and febrile illnesses. Natural killer cell function is also enhanced in children whose parents reported more chronic stress (18). Unlike older adults, children living with elevated chronic stress had enhanced rather than decreased natural killer cell functioning, suggesting that chronic stress may have different effects on the developing immune system.

Dementia caregivers have fourfold increases in the proinflammatory cytokine interleukin-6 compared with noncaregivers and have poorer health outcomes following illness (19). Even several years after the death of the impaired spouse, the changes in interleukin-6 among former caregivers did not differ from levels found in current caregivers. There were no systematic group differences in chronic health problems, medications, or health-relevant behaviors that might have accounted for the caregivers' interleukin-6 changes. Chronic stress appears to accelerate the risk of age-related diseases by prematurely aging the immune response.

Immune function, as measured by interleukin-2 and -12, plasma cortisol, and urinary catecholamines, is affected by psychological distress in patients with breast cancer and also in their adult daughters (20). Norepinephrine levels mediated the relationship between daughters' distress and their immune functions. Cortisol mediated only the relationship between daughters' distress and interleukin-2 secretion. In the daughters, stress hormone secretions and immune functions are related to both their own and their mothers' psychological distress.

The link between interpersonal relationships and immune function therefore can be seen to include diverse family and relational stressors. Disruption of relationships and the maintenance of abrasive relationships have clear effects on immune function. This research has contributed to the large literature on social relationships and health by delineating a pathway through which relationships can be beneficial or detrimental to health.

Relational Factors and the Nervous System

Regular interaction with supportive people results in diminished activity in the dorsal anterior cingulate cortex and Brodmann area 8. These regions are associated with the distress of social separation (10). These same regions and their connections through the hypothalamic-midbrain-limbic-paralimbic-cortical circuits are also involved in parents' response to their infant. Infant stimuli activate basal forebrain regions, which regulate brain circuits that handle nurturing and caregiving responses and activate the brain's general circuitry for handling emotions, motivation, attention, and empathy (21).

Monoamine oxidase A (MAO-A) activity is influenced by genetic variation. A variant of the MAO-A gene produces low MAO-A activity and is associated with antisocial behavior in maltreated boys (22). The variant of the MAO-A gene that produces high MAO-A activity is not associated with antisocial behavior in maltreated boys. Maltreatment was defined by parental reports of neglect, exposure to intraparental violence, and inconsistent discipline.

In rhesus monkeys, early caretaking environments interact with 5-HT alleles to produce monkeys at risk for behavioral problems. Infant rhesus monkeys were raised by adult female caretakers and compared with those raised by peers. An interaction with a specific allelic risk factor, the short form of the 5-HT polymorphism that affects serotonin transport, was found to confer risk for developing alcohol-seeking behaviors in juveniles and young adults (23). In humans, individuals with the short allele developed depression only when exposed to a high-risk environment such as an impoverished early caretaking relationship environment characterized by punitive or neglectful parenting (24).

Relational Factors and Medical Illnesses

Families have a powerful influence on health equal to traditional medical risk factors. Family factors influence the course of chronic medical illnesses in four main ways according to Campbell's review of the literature (25). The quality of the marital relationship is the most influential family relationship on health for adults. Emotional support is the most important and influential type of support provided by families. However, negative, critical, or hostile family relationships have a stronger influence on health than positive or supportive relationships.

Relational factors in medical illnesses

Protective factors
- Good communication
- Adaptability
- Clear roles
- Achieving family development tasks
- Supporting individual members
- Expressing appreciation
- Commitment to the family
- Religious/spiritual orientation
- Social connectedness
- Spending time together

Risk factors
- Family conflict
- Rigidity
- Blame
- High levels of criticism

The family relationships that influence disease outcome consist of protective and risk factors (26). Protective factors are present with healthy family processes. Healthy families are characterized as communicating well, encouraging individual family members, expressing appreciation, being committed to the family, having a religious or spiritual orientation, being socially connected, being adaptable, having clear roles, and spending time together. Healthy families do not allow the disease to interfere with normal family developmental tasks. Several protective factors where the evidence is suggestive of protection (but not proven) are also recognized. These factors include the ability to talk about emotional issues, the integration of ritual and routine in family life, secure attachments for children, good problem-solving ability, and family recreation time. Family risk factors include intrafamilial conflict, blame, rigidity, and high levels of criticism. Criticalness and hostility are considered the most influential risk factors on disease outcome.

Patients who act as caregivers are at increased risk for more general health problems, including influenza, upper respiratory infections, stomach disorders, headaches, back pain, sleeplessness, and depression. For example, women who care for a disabled or ill spouse for 9 or more hours per week are at increased risk of coronary artery disease (27). It is interesting to note that this association is not present when the female caregiver cares for other relatives such as a parent or child.

Evidence-Based Family Interventions and Medical Illnesses

Family interventions in medical illnesses can be aimed at health promotion, illness prevention, and intervention in the acute stage with the goal of reducing chronicity, or at later stages to help with management of chronic illness.

Family Intervention and the Promotion of Healthy Behaviors and Prevention of Illness

Risk factors for a variety of chronic medical illnesses include nicotine dependence, obesity, lack of exercise, and poor diet. All of these risk factors are the focus of intervention by health psychologists and physicians. Family treatments have been developed for many of these risk factors. For example, in an innovative smoking cessation program, smokers and nonsmoking partners are randomly assigned to either behavioral couples treatment (BCT) or a standard treatment for smoking cessation (28). The objective of this research is to improve smoking cessation rates using a manualized partner or family-involved intervention. This research is based on the successful treatment of alcohol or drug-abusing populations where BCT demonstrated significantly greater long-term abstinence rates, improved pharmacotherapy compliance, and reduced risk for relapse for up to 2 years posttreatment compared with individual-only treatment (29).

Family interventions used in medical illnesses

- Couples communication training in hypertension
- Couples therapy in chronic low back pain
- Family-focused intervention for diabetes
- Psychosocial intervention with patients with systemic lupus erythematosus and partners
- Caregiver interventions for dementia
- Palliative care discussions about end-of-life issues

Other studies that focus on promoting healthy behaviors include communication training for couples with marital conflict, which reduces blood pressure in people with essential hypertension (30), and caregiver intervention programs that focus on preventing depression and caregiver burden, thus enhancing the care of the dementia patient (31).

Family Interventions in the Acute Phase With the Purpose of Reducing Chronicity

Spouses of patients with coronary artery bypass graft (226 male and 70 female) were randomly assigned to either view or not view a psychoeducational video prior to the patient's release from the hospital. Women, whether patients or caregivers, were noted to be generally at elevated risk for negative outcome in the 6-month follow-up. However, female patients who had spouses who watched the psychoeducational tape had less risk for negative health outcome (32).

A support and education program for spouses of stroke victims improved the quality of life and general well-being for spouses. The positive impact at 12 months was only found, however, for spouses attending at least five to six times (33). Further studies need to be done to assess the impact of psychoeducational interventions over substantial periods of time and to determine if "booster" support or psychoeducational sessions might be helpful.

Family-focused approach to the management of chronic disease

- Help families manage stresses as a team
- Mobilize patient's natural support system
- Enhance family closeness
- Increase mutually supportive interactions
- Build extrafamilial support
- Minimize intrafamilial hostility and criticism
- Reduce adverse effects of external stress and disease-related trauma

Family Interventions and Management of Chronic Medical Illnesses

Chronic illness has a profound effect on family functioning. The multiple changes that families undergo when a family member has a chronic medical illness include acute coping strategies as well as long-term grieving and role reassignment (34). For most chronic illnesses, the family's ability to provide consistent illness management is crucial for optimal patient outcome.

A family-focused approach to the management of chronic disease addresses three main goals (26):

1. To help families cope with and manage the continuing stresses inherent in chronic disease management as a team rather than as individuals.

2. To mobilize the patient's natural support system to enhance family closeness, increase mutually supportive interactions among family members, and build additional extrafamilial support, with the goal of improving disease management and the health and well-being of patients and all family members.

3. To minimize intrafamilial hostility and criticism and to reduce the adverse effects of external stress and disease-related trauma on family life.

Family-focused interventions should aim to help family members agree on and collaborate with a program of disease management in ways that are consistent with their beliefs and operational style; help family members manage stress by preventing the disease from dominating family life and sacrificing normal developmental and personal goals; help the family deal with the losses that chronic illness can create; mobilize the family's natural support system to provide education and support for all family members involved in disease management; reduce social isolation and resulting anxiety and depression that disease management can create in both the patient and other family members; and reorganize the family, with adjustments of roles and expectations as needed, to ensure optimal patient self-care.

Family Intervention in the Management of Chronic Childhood Illness

Successful family interventions can be implemented in many treatment settings. At the Joslin Clinic in Boston, children and adolescents were randomly assigned to a family-focused teamwork intervention or to standard multidisciplinary diabetes care. The family-focused intervention group emphasized family teamwork, particularly in the area of insulin injections and measurement of the blood glucose. Both groups met three to four times a year. The family intervention required some, but not extensive training for the clinic staff. This low-cost family intervention reduced family conflict in adolescents, improved the management of diabetes, prevented complications, and improved family relationships, at little added expense to the clinic (35).

Couples Treatment in the Management of Chronic Adult Illness

Sixty-four adults with systemic lupus erythematosus and their partners were given a psychoeducational intervention to enhance self-efficacy, communication about lupus, social support, and problem solving. The intervention consisted of a 1-hour session with a nurse educator, followed by monthly counseling via telephone for 6 months. The control group of 55 patients and their partners received an attention placebo, which consisted of a 45-minute video presentation about lupus and monthly telephone follow-up calls for 6 months. After 1 year, the group receiving psychoeducation reported improved communication, increased levels of social support, and reduced levels of patient fatigue, compared with the control group (36).

Patients with chronic low back pain participated in a controlled, prospective study to evaluate the long-term effects of five-session couples therapy (37). At the 5-year follow-up assessments, psychological distress was less in the treatment group with no difference in marital satisfaction, health locus of control, pain, or disability. Couples therapy has a prolonged beneficial effect on the mental well-being of patients with chronic lower back pain, although this did not translate into improved health care outcome.

Family Intervention in the Management of Chronic Adult Illness

Palliative care is the interdisciplinary specialty that aims to relieve suffering and improve the quality of care for patients with serious illness and their families. Palliative care integrates the needs of the family into the care of the patient, needs determined by the family as they attend to the care of their dying relative. Telephone interviews were conducted with 190 family members of patients who had died, to assess the family's satisfaction with the quality of medical care at the end of life. Those family members of patients who had received palliative care showed benefit, with 65% of palliative-care patients' family members reporting that their emotional or spiritual needs were met, as compared with 35% of usual-care patients' family members ($P<0.004$) (38). Among palliative-care patients' family members, 67% reported greater self-efficacy, as compared with 44% of usual-care patients' family members. Palliative care offers a unique approach by integrating the needs of the family into the care of the patient without the use of specific protocols.

Relational Factors and Psychiatric Illnesses

Discussion of family factors in psychiatric illness has a long and checkered history. As early as 1934, Kasanin had suggested that parenting problems such as maternal rejection or overprotection were influential in causing schizophrenia. Fromm-Reichmann (39) stated that "the schizophrenic is painfully distrustful and resentful of other people due to the severe early warp and rejection he encountered in important people in his infancy and childhood, as a rule mainly the schizophrenogenic mother" (p. 265). Uncontrolled studies developed concepts such as marital schism and marital skew to explain schizophrenia in the child (40). Family systems theorists continued the preoccupation with the dysfunctional family, developing other concepts such as the double-bind theory of schizophrenia (41), which involved disordered communications within the family unit, with the mother as the most disordered family member. Donald Jackson (42) wrote that "perhaps the next phase will include a study of schizophrenia as a family borne disease involving a complicated host-vector recipient cycle that includes much more than can be connoted by the term, schizophrenogenic mother. One could even speculate whether schizophrenia as it is known today would exist if parthenogenesis was the usual mode of propagation of the human species or if women were impersonally impregnated and gave birth to infants who were reared by state nurses in a communal setting" (p. 184). These theories were put forward without research to back them up and have since proved not only erroneous but highly damaging to families doing the best they can to deal with their sick relative.

Current psychiatric practice may inadvertently perpetuate the perception that bad parents are the cause of psychiatric illness by focusing exclusively on the experience of the patient. Gunderson (43) reported that he was surprised when he met the parents of patients with borderline personality disorder and found them to be reasonable people, stating that he had been duped into believing what the patients had said about their families. It is therefore important for all psychiatrists to guard against unsubstantiated bias against families.

Relational factors in psychiatric illnesses

Protective factors
- Low expressed emotion
- Emotional overinvolvement for borderline personality disorder

Risk factors
- Relationship discord
- High expressed emotion
- High caregiver burden
- Poor social support

Relational Dysfunction/Marital Conflict and Psychiatric Illness

Relational dysfunction or discord causes psychological distress and is associated with increased risk for mood disorders, anxiety disorders, and substance use disorders (44). Couples interviewed in the National Comorbidity Study were assessed for relationship discord with two questions: "All in all, how satisfied are you with your relationship—very, somewhat, not very, or not at all satisfied?" and "Overall, would you rate your relationship as excellent, good, fair, or poor?" Individuals ($n=2,766$) in discordant relationships reported greater social role impairment with relatives and friends, greater work role impairment, higher levels of general distress, poorer perceived health, and more reported suicidal ideation. With the exception of suicidal ideation, the associations between relationship discord and impairment and psychological distress remained significant after controlling for current mood, anxiety, and substance use disorders, suggesting that relationship discord is incrementally related to impairment and psychological distress over and above the effects of psychiatric disorders.

Marital discord is reported as a risk factor for suicide attempts in African American women (45), and low levels of social support in general are associated with suicide ideation (46). Marital discord also has an impact on parenting ability (47) and childhood illness (see above sections on relational factors and the immune system/endocrine system). For example, alcoholism in a parent negatively affects childhood functioning, which then improves with the treatment of the parent's illness. Before their fathers' treatment, children exhibited greater symptomatology than children from the matched sample and improved significantly following their fathers' treatment. Children of stably remitted fathers were similar to their peers from the control group and had fewer adjustment problems than children of relapsed fathers, even after accounting for children's baseline adjustment (48).

Greater marital discord is found in people with specific psychiatric disorders, including depression (49) and panic disorder (50), but the direction of causality is unclear. In a large population-based community sample from Ontario, Canada, people with a current psychiatric disorder were more likely to report troubled relationships with their spouse than people without a disorder, 24.5% and 8.9%, respectively (51). Regardless of which comes first, the problems coexist and both are worthy of treatment.

Recovery from illness is often slower when family dysfunction is present. Patients with major depression have a slower rate of recovery when they live in families with significant family dysfunction (52). Patients with good family functioning at the time of hospitalization generally maintain their healthy functioning and are more likely to recover by 12 months than patients with poor family functioning (53). Good family functioning is one of five factors that is associated with a good outcome in major depression (54). Family treatment therefore can be of major benefit in obtaining recovery from illness. The enclosed DVD shows a family in which the identified patient is the wife/mother with long-standing depressive symptoms. The associated family dysfunction is assessed and family treatment initiated. **The impact of the depression on the family is shown in scene 4. The formulation of the interplay between the depression and the family is presented to the family in scene 13.**

Expressed emotion (EE) is the family construct that has been most studied and researched worldwide. In the 1950s, George Brown and his colleagues at the Social Research Unit in London noticed that patients with schizophrenia were more likely to relapse if they returned to live with parents or spouses than if they went to live in lodgings or with siblings (55). The researchers hypothesized that the close emotional ties of family life overstimulated the patients with schizophrenia, who then became withdrawn and isolated in an attempt to reduce their level of social contact. EE measures criticism, hostility, and emotional overinvolvement in families. High-EE families make more critical and hostile comments during a family interview. Criticisms are defined as comments about the behavior or characteristics of the patient, which the respondent clearly resents or is annoyed by. Hostility is rated categorically, according to whether the respondent makes generalized criticisms of the patient, expresses attitudes that are rejecting of the patient, neither of these, or both. Scores for emotional overinvolvement and warmth are assigned by the rater after taking into account comments made and attitudes expressed throughout the interview; the score is a composite measure of factors such as an exaggerated emotional response, overintrusive or self-sacrificing behavior, and overidentification with the patient. Although initially used with schizophrenic patients and their families, EE is now studied extensively across the health care spectrum and in many cultures (56).

For patients with schizophrenia, living in a high-EE family confers a relapse rate of three to four times, compared with living in a low-EE family (57).

For patients with bipolar disorder, living in a high-EE family confers a relapse rate to a depressive episode five times that of living in a low-EE family (58). At first analysis, the Miklowitz Colorado Treatment/Outcome Project did not find this rate of relapse. However, when the patients' symptom severity was assessed, rather than their relapse status, patients from high-EE families had significantly higher levels of depression compared with patients from low-EE families (59). Patients with major depression also show high relapse rates and relapse at relatively low levels of criticism when they live with high-EE relatives (60). Two or more critical comments are associated with relapse for patients with major depression, compared with six or more critical comments associated with relapse for patients with schizophrenia (61). Typically, family members of patients with major depression make at least seven critical remarks (60, 61). Lower ratings of EE are found when the patient is elderly, with only four to five critical comments; the highest ratings occur in patients who have recurrent or chronic illnesses (62). Having a partner who is consistently uncritical or who is critical only at presentation is associated with the best prognosis for major depression (63). Patients with alcohol dependency are more likely to relapse, have a shorter time to relapse, and drink on a greater percentage of days if they have high-EE spouses rather than low-EE spouses. EE is associated with relapse even after patients' age, education, and severity of alcohol problem are taken into account (64). Children with obsessive-compulsive disorder often live in families with high EE (65). High EE is also a strong predictor of poor outcome for patients with eating disorders and obesity (66). On the other hand, high levels of emotional overinvolvement are associated with a lower probability of hospital readmissions among patients with borderline personality disorder after 12 months (67).

Other Family Factors That Affect Course and Outcome in Psychiatric Illnesses

Negative life events and poor social support are associated with more depressive symptoms and depression recurrences in bipolar disorder (20). A recent study of families of patients with bipolar disorder attempts to link three concepts: caregiver burden, emotional overinvolvement (a component of EE), and patient outcome. Families who experience the highest burden in caring for their relative show the highest emotional overinvolvement, and these patients have poor adherence to their medication regimes resulting in an increased likelihood to relapse (68). The family members' experience of burden was not affected by the severity of symptoms or whether they lived with the patient. However, burden was significantly associated with the family's perception of stigma regarding psychiatric illness.

In summary, good relational factors improve life trajectories. Good marital relationships in adult lives improve the trajectories of boys identified as delinquent in their younger years (69) and in women who were previously diagnosed with borderline personality disorder (70). Although what constitutes "good" marital relationships may not be clearly defined, the researchers in these studies suggest factors such as emotional support, affirmation such as the expression of empathy, warmth, and genuineness, as well as relationships that provide specific needed factors (e.g., assertiveness vs. passivity). Parenting style and marital quality are thus well recognized in the development of health, whereas deficiencies in these areas are now being shown to contribute to medical and psychiatric illness.

Evidence-based family interventions for psychiatric illnesses

- Alcohol dependence: **behavioral couples therapy**
- Prevention of PTSD in children, siblings, and parents: **SCCIP**
- Prevention of schizophrenia: **early-intervention programs**
- Schizophrenia: **psychoeducational multifamily groups**
- Bipolar disorder: **IFIT, PCSTF, FFT**
- Major depression: **behavioral couples therapy, PCSTF**
- Borderline personality disorder: **multifamily treatment**
- Conduct disorder: **family therapy**
- ADHD in children: **family therapy**
- Depression and anxiety in children: **family therapy**
- Eating disorders in adolescents and adults: **family therapy**
- Obsessive-compulsive disorder in children: **family therapy**

ADHD=attention-deficit/hyperactivity disorder; FFT=family-focused therapy; IFIT=integrated family and individual therapy; PCSTF=Problem-Centered Systems Therapy of the Family; PTSD=posttraumatic stress disorder; SCCIP=Surviving Cancer Competently Intervention Program.

Evidence-Based Family Interventions and Psychiatric Illnesses

Family Intervention: The Promotion of Healthy Behaviors and Prevention of Illness

Family members benefit indirectly from treatment of the identified patient. Children of alcoholics show significantly improved psychosocial adjustment after their fathers enter treatment (48). Intimate partner violence is reduced when alcohol dependence is treated with behavioral couples therapy (BCT) (71). In one study, couples-based therapy was compared with individual-based therapy for men who entered outpatient substance abuse treatment. Men were randomly assigned to 1) BCT, 2) individual-based treatment, or 3) couples-based psychoeducational attention control treatment. For both children of alcohol-abusing ($n=71$) and drug-abusing ($n=64$) men, parents' ratings of children's psychosocial functioning were higher for children whose fathers participated in BCT at 6- and 12-month follow-ups. BCT also resulted in greater improvements in parents' dyadic adjustment and fathers' substance use (72).

Posttraumatic stress disorder can be prevented in young adult survivors of childhood cancer and their family members (73). The Surviving Cancer Competently Intervention Program integrates cognitive-behavioral and family therapy approaches in a 1-day program. Significant reductions in intrusive thoughts among fathers and in arousal among survivors were found in the treatment group. The data are supportive of brief interventions for multiple members of the family.

Family Interventions in the Acute Phase With the Purpose of Reducing Chronicity

Recent interest in schizophrenia focuses on the prevention of the initial episode or early intervention. Psychoeducational multifamily group treatment has been proposed as part of early treatment programs. However, patients and families often have to wait for sufficient numbers before a group can start. Treatment is generally well received by patients and families, but no evidence is yet available to tell if this is successful in reducing the incidence or improving the course of schizophrenia (74).

Family Intervention in Management of Chronic Childhood Illness

Family intervention for children with obsessive-compulsive disorder (OCD) is superior to individual therapy (75). In a study of 28 patients with treatment-refractory OCD, the family participated in an 8-week psychoeducational group designed to reduce accommodation to OCD symptoms. Multifamily group treatment for OCD compares favorably with individual family therapy in children and adolescents (76). Group family treatment uses a cognitive-behavioral protocol, with additional parental and sibling components. The family component focuses on managing the child's OCD and teaching parents and siblings strategies to manage their own distress. Parent sessions focus on psychoeducation and problem-solving skills and strategies to reduce parental involvement in the child's symptoms, along with encouraging family support of home-based exposure and response prevention trials. The program emphasizes that coping strategies need to be practiced as a family on a daily basis. This protocol provides an example of a well-designed psychoeducational program that can be implemented in conjunction with the individual treatment of the child or adolescent.

Couples Treatment in Management of Chronic Adult Illness

Couples and family treatment used in research has to be manualized for standardization and replication. Therefore psychoeducational or interventions based on cognitive-behavioral therapy are more commonly used. Couples therapy is particularly helpful when marital distress is present.

BCT has been shown to be effective in the treatment of major depression (77, 78). In general, behavioral marital therapy is comparable with individual therapy in improving depressive symptoms and better than individual therapy in improving marital functioning. In addition, outpatients with mild to moderate major depression report that couples therapy is preferable to antidepressant medication (79). In this study, 77 outpatients and their partners were randomly assigned to couples therapy or to either desipramine or a selective serotonin reuptake inhibitor and were followed for 1 year. The couples therapy, delivered over 12–20 sessions, consisted of interventions such as the interruption of problematic transactions and the setting of tasks.

BCT is more effective than individual treatment at increasing abstinence from alcohol, improving relationship functioning, and limiting emotional problems in the children of participants (80). However, BCT is intensive and requires a time commitment of up to 22 sessions over 6 months. Following those initial sessions are 10 to 12 weekly conjoint pregroup sessions with each couple, followed by 10 two-hour multifamily groups. BCT also implements a Daily Sobriety Contract that includes administration of Antabuse under spousal supervision.

Family Intervention in Management of Chronic Adult Illness

Schizophrenia is the psychiatric illness in which family intervention has been most studied. The provision of family psychoeducation reduces patient relapse rate to 15% per year compared with 30%–40% for patients who do not receive this intervention. Improving family coping skills was one of the main goals of the first psychoeducation interventions for families with a relative with schizophrenia (81). Family psychoeducation for schizophrenia is based on the premise that the patient has a brain disorder and that families need to be supported in their care of the mentally ill person. The emphasis on the biological aspect of the illness is intended to correct the misperception that families somehow cause the illness. This unfortunate misperception originated in early work with patients with schizophrenia and their families. The most frequent components of psychoeducational programs are problem-focused skills training, positive communication development, and increased social involvement for the family. Family psychoeducation includes the provision of emotional support, illness education, and resources during periods of crisis. Emphasis is placed on families learning from each other, as mutual support is considered to be one of the main therapeutic factors in these programs (see box) (82).

However, Mexican immigrants who received behavioral family therapy actually relapsed at a higher rate than patients who received traditional case management (83). In Spain, no difference in patient relapse rate was found between patients whose families participated in psychoeducational programs compared with families in the control group (84). It is therefore unclear if there are specific culturally dependent family needs. The needs and preferences of family members of adults with mental illness are diverse, and families may benefit best from intervention tailored to meet families' individual needs. Continued efforts should be made to understand and address family needs, potential barriers to participation in family services, and the relationship between stigma and family needs.

Family interventions used in
chronic adult illness

- Coordinate care with all providers
- Attend to social needs of family
- Provide optimal medication management
- Listen to families and treat them as equal partners in treatment planning and delivery
- Explore family members' expectations of treatment and for the patient
- Assess family's strengths and limitations in being able to support the patient
- Help resolve family conflict
- Address feelings of loss
- Provide relevant information at appropriate times
- Provide explicit crisis plan
- Improve communication and problem solving
- Encourage family to expand social network
- Be flexible in meeting the family's needs

Source.   Adapted from McFarlane et al. 2003 (82).

Family interventions for bipolar disorder have yielded mixed results. This is due in part to the nature of the illness, as patients can do well for intermittent periods but still have an unfavorable long-term course. It is also hard to compare results from various family therapy studies because of differences in the types of treatment provided and ways in which the treatments are delivered. For example, family treatments can last 6–8 sessions over 2–6 months or 25+ sessions over 12 months. Some studies use only one therapist whereas some use cotherapists; some family therapies are provided in a multifamily group format and others as single family therapy. Despite these limitations, studies suggest that adjunctive family interventions are useful in modifying family functioning and the course of bipolar disorder (85, 86).

Family-focused therapy helps patients avoid rehospitalization during symptomatic deterioration. In one study, patients with bipolar disorder who received family-focused therapy were rehospitalized at a rate of 12% compared with the control group rate of 60% (87). In a related study that combined integrated family and individual therapy with mood-stabilizing pharmacotherapy, patients went a longer time without relapsing than those receiving case management (42.5 vs. 34.5 weeks) (88).

For patients from families with high levels of impairment, the addition of a family intervention results in an improved course of illness (89). In contrast, for patients from families with low impairment, the addition of the family intervention does not improve the course of illness. This study used a multifamily group therapy psychoeducational treatment consisting of four to six families (including the patient) who met for six sessions with cotherapists plus single family therapy. Improvement in family functioning was independent of symptomatic improvement in the patient. The addition of family therapy resulted in lower rehospitalization rates when patients relapsed, suggesting that families had learned how to deal more effectively with recurrences (90).

Family therapy is a useful adjunct to pharmacotherapy for patients with depression, particularly when the depression is severe or when the depressive episode evolves in a social context characterized by marital/family distress. The effectiveness of the Problem-Centered Systems Therapy of the Family was evaluated in a study of 121 patients who were randomly assigned to pharmacotherapy alone, combined pharmacotherapy and cognitive therapy, combined pharmacotherapy and family therapy, or combined pharmacotherapy, cognitive therapy and family therapy (91). The addition of family treatment to pharmacotherapy and/or cognitive therapy led to greater proportions of patients who improved and to significantly greater reductions in depression and suicidal ideation.

Multifamily groups treatment is also useful for families who have a relative with borderline personality disorder. It was assumed that the families of borderline patients were "overinvolved, separation-resistant with dependency generating mothers" but when these families were actually studied, they were found to be underinvolved (43). These families identified problems with communication, conflict, and anger and difficulty managing the patient's suicidality. Multifamily groups focused on looking toward the future and learning new coping strategies. The first phase of treatment consisted of joining session(s), and the second phase consisted of multifamily group treatment lasting approximately 18 months. Results of the family treatment included increased communication and decreased family conflict.

Adolescents with anorexia nervosa benefit from family therapy, especially when parents take an active role with the adolescent (92). Single family therapy and multifamily psychoeducation groups are equally effective in weight restoration (93). In adults with anorexia nervosa, family therapy is comparable with individual psychotherapy, and both are superior to a control group (94).

Conclusion

The validity of family-based interventions is recognized by the American Psychiatric Association's Practice Guidelines. The second edition of the guidelines for schizophrenia (95) outlines in detail the importance of involving the family in management of the illness and recognizes different interventions for different stages of the illness. During an acute episode, the guidelines recommend establishing a therapeutic alliance with the family and addressing the family's needs. The guidelines recommend routinely meeting with family members to obtain information and to provide information on the management of the illness. They state: "Educational meetings and survival workshops that teach families how to cope with schizophrenia and referrals to local chapters of patient and family organizations such as NAMI [National Alliance on Mental Illness] may be helpful and are recommended. Families may be under considerable stress, particularly if the patient has been exhibiting dangerous or unstable behavior" (p. 5).

During the stable phase, the guidelines recommend educating the family about signs of relapse and advising them to develop a plan of action should these signs appear. The guidelines recommend that family members receive support, problem-solving training, and communication training. The role of family members in helping with medication compliance is emphasized, and the provision of manuals, workbooks, and videotapes for family members is recommended. The efficacy of family interventions in preventing relapse and improving patient functioning and family well-being is emphasized. The guidelines state: "On the basis of the evidence, persons with schizophrenia and their families who have ongoing contact with each other should be offered a family intervention, the key elements of which include a duration of at least 9 months, illness education, crisis intervention, emotional support and training in how to cope with illness symptoms and related problems" (p. 35).

The practice guidelines for bipolar disorder (96) and major depression (97) recommend early family involvement and present the efficacy of family-based interventions. Practice guidelines for other disorders such as panic disorder, eating disorders, and substance abuse disorders similarly recommend early involvement of the family and provide evidence of the marital or family therapy as psychosocial interventions.

References

1. Tienari P, Wynne LC, Sorri A, et al: Genotype-environment interaction in schizophrenia-spectrum disorder: long-term follow-up study of Finnish adoptees. Br J Psychiatry 184:216–222, 2004
2. Reiss D, Neirderhiser JM: The interplay of genetic influences and social processes in developmental theory: specific mechanisms are coming into view. Dev Psychopathol 12:357–374, 2000
3. Cadoret RJ, Winokur G, Langbehn D, et al: Depression spectrum disease, I: the role of gene-environment interaction. Am J Psychiatry 153:892–899, 1996
4. Coyne JC, Rohrbaugh MJ, Shoham V, et al: Prognostic importance of marital quality for survival of congestive heart failure. Am J Cardiol 88:526–529, 2001
5. Berkman L, Leo-Summers L, Horowitz RI: Emotional support and survival after myocardial infarction. Ann Intern Med 117:1003–1009, 1992
6. Rohrbaugh MJ, Shoham V, Coyne JC: Effect of marital quality on eight-year survival of patients with heart failure. Am J Cardiol 98:1069–1072, 2006
7. Gallo LC, Troxel WM, Matthews KA, et al: Marital status and quality in middle-aged women: associations with levels and trajectories of cardiovascular risk factors. Health Psychol 22:453–463, 2003
8. Kiecolt-Glaser JK, Newton TL: Marriage and health: his and hers. Psychol Bull 127:472–503, 2001
9. Flinn MV, England BG: Social economics of childhood glucocorticoid stress response and health. Am J Phys Anthropol 102:33–53, 1997
10. Eisenberger NI, Taylor SE, Gable SL, et al: Neural pathways link social support to attenuated neuroendocrine stress responses. Neuroimage 35:1601–1612, 2007
11. Shannon C, Schwandt ML, Champoux M, et al: Maternal absence and stability of individual differences in CSF 5-HIAA concentrations in rhesus monkey infants. Am J Psychiatry 162:1658–1664, 2005
12. Erickson K, Gabry KE, Lindell S, et al: Social withdrawal behaviors in nonhuman primates and changes in neuroendocrine and monoamine concentrations during a separation paradigm. Dev Psychobiol 46:331–339, 2005

13. Francis DD, Young LJ, Meaney MJ, et al: Naturally occurring differences in maternal care are associated with the expression of oxytocin and vasopressin (VIa) receptors: gender differences. J Neuroendocrinol 14:349–353, 2002
14. Heinrichs M, Baumgartner T, Kirschbaum C, et al: Social support and oxytocin interact to suppress cortisol and subjective responses to psychosocial stress. Biol Psychiatry 54:1389–1398, 2003
15. Ross LE, Sellers EM, Gilbert Evans SE, et al: Mood changes during pregnancy and the post-partum period: development of a biopsychosocial model. Acta Psychiatr Scand 109:457–466, 2004
16. Kiecolt-Glaser JK, McGuire L, Robles TF, et al: Psychoneuroimmunology and psychosomatic medicine: back to the future. Psychosom Med 64:15–20, 2002
17. Glaser R, Robles TF, Sheridan J, et al: Mild depressive symptoms are associated with amplified and prolonged inflammatory responses after influenza virus vaccination in older adults. Arch Gen Psychiatry 60:1009–1014, 2003
18. Wyman PA, Moynihan J, Eberly S, et al: Association of family stress with natural killer cell activity and the frequency of illnesses in children. Arch Pediatr Adolesc Med 161:228–234, 2007
19. Kiecolt-Glaser JK, Preacher KJ, MacCullum RC, et al: Chronic stress and age-related increases in the proinflammatory cytokine IL-6. Proc Natl Acad Sci USA 100:9090–9095, 2003
20. Cohen AN, Hammen C, Henry RM, et al: Effects of stress and social support on recurrence in bipolar disorder. J Affect Disord 82:143–147, 2004
21. Swain JE, Lorberbaum JP, Kose S, et al: Brain basis of early parent-infant interactions: psychology, physiology, and in vivo functional neuroimaging studies. J Child Psychol Psychiatry 48:262–287, 2007
22. Kim-Cohen J, Caspi A, Taylor A, et al: MAOA, maltreatment, and gene-environment interaction predicting children's mental health: new evidence and a meta-analysis. Mol Psychiatry 11:903–913, 2006
23. Barr CS, Newman TK, Lindell S, et al: Interaction between serotonin transporter gene variation and rearing condition in alcohol preference and consumption in female primates. Arch Gen Psychiatry 61:1146–1152, 2004
24. Caspi A, Sugden K, Moffitt TE, et al: Influence of life stress on depression: moderation by a polymorphism in the 5-HTT gene. Science 301:386–389, 2003
25. Campbell TL: The effectiveness of family interventions for physical disorders. J Marital Fam Ther 29:263–281, 2003
26. Weihs K, Fisher L, Baird MA: Families, health, and behavior: a section of the commissioned report by the Committee on Health and Behavior. Fam Syst Health 20:7–47, 2002

27. Lee S, Colditz GA, Berkman L, et al: Caregiving and risk of coronary heart disease in US women: a prospective study. Am J Prev Med 24:113–119, 2003
28. LaChance H: Behavioral couples therapy for smoking cessation: treatment development, in T. O'Farrell (Chair), Behavioral Couples Therapy for Addictive Disorders: New Applications. Paper presented at the 41st meeting of the Association for Behavioral and Cognitive Therapies, Philadelphia, PA, November 2007
29. O'Farrell TJ, Fals-Stewart W: Behavioral couples therapy for alcoholism and drug abuse. J Subst Abuse Treat 18:51–54, 2000
30. Ewart CK, Taylor CB, Kraemer HC, et al: High blood pressure and marital discord: not being nasty matters more than being nice. Health Psychol 10:155–163, 1991
31. Mittelman M: Taking care of the caregivers. Curr Opin Psychiatry 18:633–639, 2005
32. Mahler HI, Kulik JA: Effects of a videotape information intervention for spouses on spouse distress and patient recovery from surgery. Health Psychol 21:427–437, 2002
33. Larson J, Franzen-Dahlin A, Billing E, et al: The impact of a nurse-led support and education programme for spouses of stroke patients: a randomized controlled trial. J Clin Nurs 14:995–1003, 2005
34. Rolland JS: Families, Illness and Disability: An Integrative Treatment Model. New York, Basic Books, 1994
35. Laffel L, Vangsness L, Connell A, et al: Impact of ambulatory, family focused teamwork intervention on glycemic control in youth with type 1 diabetes. J Pediatr 142:409–416, 2003
36. Karlson EW, Liang MH, Eaton H, et al: A randomized clinical trial of a psychoeducational intervention to improve outcomes in systemic lupus erythematosus. Arthritis Rheum 50:1832–1841, 2004
37. Saarijarvi S, Alanen E, Rytokoski U, et al: Couple therapy improves marital wellbeing in chronic low back pain patients: a controlled five-year follow-up study. J Psychosom Res 36:651–656, 1992
38. Gelfman LP, Meier DE, Morrison RS: Does palliative care improve quality? A survey of bereaved family members. J Pain Symptom Manage 36:22–28, 2008
39. Fromm-Reichmann F: Notes on the development of the treatment of schizophrenics by psychoanalytic psychotherapy. Psychiatry 11:263–273, 1948
40. Lidz T, Cornelison AR, Fleck S: The intrafamilial environment of the schizophrenic patient, part 2: marital schism and marital skew. Am J Psychiatry 114:241–248, 1957
41. Bateson GB, Jackson D, Haley JJ, et al: Towards the theory of schizophrenia. Behav Sci 1:251–264,1956

42. Jackson DD: A note on the importance of trauma in the genesis of schizophrenia. Psychiatry 20:181–184, 1957
43. Gunderson JG, Berkowitz C, Ruiz-Sancho A: Families of borderline patients: a psychoeducational approach. Bull Menninger Clin 61:446–457, 1997
44. Whisman MA, Uebelacker LA: Impairment and distress associated with relationship discord in a national sample of married or cohabiting adults. J Fam Psychol 20:369–377, 2006
45. Kaslow N, Thompson M, Meadows L, et al: Risk factors for suicide attempts among African American women. Depress Anxiety 12:13–20, 2000
46. Gunnel D, Harbord R, Singleton N, et al: Factors influencing the development and amelioration of suicidal thoughts in the general population: cohort study. Behav Ther 32:803–820, 2004
47. Cummings EM, Davies PT: Effects of marital conflict on children: recent advances and emerging themes in process-oriented research. J Child Psychol Psychiatry 43:31–63, 2002
48. Andreas JB, O'Farrell TJ, Fals-Stewart W: Does individual treatment for alcoholic fathers benefit their children? A longitudinal assessment. J Consult Clin Psychol 74:191–198, 2006
49. Weissman MM: Advances in psychiatric epidemiology: rates and risks for major depression. Am J Public Health 77:445–451, 1987
50. Markowitz JS, Weissman MM, Ouellette R, et al: Quality of life in panic disorder. Arch Gen Psychiatry 46:984–992, 1989
51. Goering P, Lin E, Campbell D, et al: Psychiatric disability in Ontario. Can J Psychiatry 41:564–571, 1996
52. Keitner GI, Miller IW: Family functioning and major depression: an overview. Am J Psychiatry 147:1128–1137, 1990
53. Keitner GI, Ryan CE, Miller IW, et al: Role of the family in recovery and major depression. Am J Psychiatry 152:1002–1008, 1995
54. Keitner GI, Ryan CE, Miller IW, et al: Recovery and major depression factors associated with twelve-month outcome. Am J Psychiatry 149:93–99, 1992
55. Brown GW, Carstairs GM, Topping G: Post-hospital adjustment of chronic mental patients. Lancet ii:685–689, 1958
56. Wearden AJ, Tarrier N, Barrowclough C, et al: A review of expressed emotion research in health care. Clin Psychol Rev 20:633–666, 2000
57. Parker G, Hadz-Pavolvic D: Expressed emotion as a predictor of schizophrenic relapse: an analysis of aggregated data. Psychol Med 20:961–965, 1990
58. Yan LJ, Hammen C, Cohen AN, et al: Expressed emotion versus relationship quality variables in the prediction of recurrence in bipolar patients. J Affect Disord 83:199–206, 2004

59. Miklowitz DJ: The role of the family in the course and treatment of bipolar disorder. Curr Dir Psychol Sci 16:192–196, 2007

60. Hooley JM: Expressed emotion and depression: interactions between patients and high- versus low-expressed-emotion spouses. J Abnorm Psychol 95:237–246, 1986

61. Vaughn CE, Leff JR: The influence of family and social factors on the course of psychiatric illness: a comparison of schizophrenic and depressed patients. Br J Psychiatry 129:125–137, 1976

62. Hinrichsen GA, Adelstein L, McMeniman M: Expressed emotion in family members of depressed older adults. Aging Ment Health 8:355–363, 2004

63. Hayhurst H, Cooper Z, Vearnals S, et al: Expressed emotion and depression: a longitudinal study. Br J Psychiatry 171:439–443, 1997

64. O'Farrell TJ, Hooley JM, Fals-Stewart W, et al: Expressed emotion and relapse in alcoholic patients. J Consult Clin Psychol 66:744–752, 1998

65. Hibbs ED, Hamburger SD, Lenane M, et al: Determinants of expressed emotion in family members of disturbed and normal children. J Child Psychol Psychiatry 32:757–770, 1991

66. van Furth EF, van Strien DC, Martina LM, et al: Expressed emotion and the prediction of outcome in adolescent eating disorders. Int J Eating Disord 20:19–31, 1996

67. Hooley JM, Hoffman PD: Expressed emotion and clinical outcome in borderline personality disorder. Am J Psychiatry 156:1557–1562, 1999

68. Perlick DA, Miklowitz DJ, Link BG, et al: Perceived stigma and depression among caregivers of patients with bipolar disorder. Br J Psychiatry 190:535–536, 2007

69. Laub J, Sampson R: Crime in the Making. Cambridge, MA, Harvard University Press, 1994

70. Paris J, Braverman S: Successful and unsuccessful marriages in borderline patients. J Am Acad Psychoanal 23:153–166, 1995

71. O'Farrell TJ, Fals-Stewart W, Murphy CM, et al: Partner violence before and after couples-based alcoholism treatment for male alcoholic patients: the role of treatment involvement and abstinence. J Consult Clin Psychol 72:202–217, 2004

72. Kelley ML, Fals-Stewart W: Couples- versus individual-based therapy for alcohol and drug abuse: effects on children's psychosocial functioning. J Consult Clin Psychol 70:417–427, 2002

73. Kazek AE, Alderfer MA, Streisand R, et al: Treatment of post traumatic stress symptoms in adolescent survivors of childhood cancer and their families: a randomized clinical trial. J Fam Psychol 18:493–504, 2004

74. Fjell A, Bloch Thorsen GR, Friis S, et al: Multifamily group treatment in a program for patients with first-episode psychosis: experiences from TIPS project. Psychiatr Serv 58:171–173, 2007

75. Grunes MS, Neziroglu F, McKay D: Family involvement in the behavioral treatment of obsessive-compulsive disorder: a preliminary investigation. Behav Therapy 32:803–820, 2001

76. Barrett P, Healy Farrell L, March JS: Cognitive-behavioral family treatment of childhood obsessive-compulsive disorder: a controlled trial. J Am Acad Child Adolesc Psychiatry 43:46–62, 2004

77. Jacobson NS, Dobson K, Fruzzetti AE, et al: Marital therapy as a treatment for depression. J Consult Clin Psychol 59:547–557, 1991

78. O'Leary KD, Beach SRH: Marital therapy: a viable treatment for depression and marital discord. Am J Psychiatry 147:183–186, 1990

79. Leff J, Vearnals S, Wolff G, et al: The London Depression Intervention Trial: randomized controlled trial of antidepressants v. couple therapy in the treatment and maintenance of people with depression living with a partner: clinical outcome and costs. Br J Psychiatry 177:95–100, 2000

80. O'Farrell T, Fals-Stewart W: Alcohol abuse. J Marital Fam Ther 29:121–146, 2003

81. Anderson CM, Hogarty GE, Reiss DJ: Family treatment of adult schizophrenic patients: a psychoeducational approach. Schizophr Bull 65:490–505, 1980

82. MacFarlane WR, Dixon L, Lukens E, et al: Family psychoeducation and schizophrenia: a review of the literature. J Marital Fam Ther 29:223–245, 2003

83. Telles C, Karno M, Mintz J, et al: Immigrant families coping with schizophrenia: behavioral family intervention vs. case management with a low-income Spanish-speaking population. Br J Psychiatry 167:473–479, 1995

84. Canive JM, Sanz-Fuentenebro J, Vazque C, et al: Family psychoeducational support groups in Spain: parents' distress and burden at one-month follow-up. Ann Clin Psychiatry 8: 71–79, 1996

85. Glick ID, Clarklin JF, Spencer JH, et al: A controlled evaluation of inpatient family interventions. Arch Gen Psychiatry 42:882–886, 1985

86. Retzer A, Simon FB, Weber G, et al: A follow-up study of manic-depressive and schizoaffective psychoses after systemic family therapy. Fam Process 30:139–153, 1991

87. Rea MM, Tompson MC, Miklowitz FJ, et al: Family-focused treatment versus individual treatment for bipolar disorder: results of a randomized clinical trial. J Consult Clin Psychol 71:482–492, 2003

88. Miklowitz DJ, Richards JA, Frank E, et al: Integrated family and individual therapy for bipolar disorder: results of a treatment development study. J Clin Psychiatry 64:182–191, 2003

89. Miller IW, Keitner GI, Ryan CE, et al: Family treatment for bipolar disorder: family impairment by treatment interactions. J Clin Psychiatry 69:732–740, 2008

90. Solomon DA, Keitner GI, Ryan CE, et al: Preventing recurrence of bipolar 1 mood episodes and hospitalizations: family psychotherapy plus pharmacotherapy alone. Bipolar Disord 10:798–805, 2008

91. Miller IW, Keitner GI, Ryan CE, et al: Treatment matching in the post hospital care of depressed patients. Am J Psychiatry 162:2131–2138, 2005

92. Asen E: Outcome research in family therapy. Adv Psychiatr Treat 8:230–238, 2002

93. Geist R, Heinman M, Stephens D, et al: Comparison of family therapy and family group psychoeducation in adolescents with anorexia nervosa. Can J Psychiatry 45:173–178, 2000

94. Dare C, Eisler I, Russell G, et al: Psychological therapies for adults with anorexia nervosa: randomized controlled trial of outpatient treatments. Br J Psychiatry 178:216–221, 2001

95. American Psychiatric Association Work Group on Schizophrenia: Practice guideline for the treatment of patients with schizophrenia, 2nd edition. Am J Psychiatry 161 (2 suppl):1–56, 2004

96. American Psychiatric Association Work Group on Bipolar Disorder: Practice guideline for the treatment of patients with bipolar disorder (revision). Am J Psychiatry 159 (4 suppl):1–50, 2002

97. American Psychiatric Association Work Group on Depressive Disorder: Practice guideline for the treatment of patients with depressive disorder (revision). Am J Psychiatry 157 (4 suppl):1–45, 2000

4

Family Assessment

- Family assessment is an essential step in developing a biopsycho-social treatment plan.
- Some family models help clinicians complete comprehensive family assessments.
- Family assessment does not necessarily lead to family therapy.
- Family assessments should be broad-based and not focused on a few family functions.
- It is desirable to have as many family members as possible present for an assessment.
- Family assessment instruments are available.

The essential task in meeting with the family members for the first time in family assessment is to evaluate and assess their functioning in the context of understanding their "problem." The family assessment is the first step in determining both the need for further interventions and the specific areas of family life that might need to be addressed. Data from the family assessment provide evidence for developing a formulation that addresses both the patients' problems and the social context in which they present. The formulation, in turn, should lead to a treatment plan that includes dealing with the biological, psychological, and social components of the problem. The family assessment provides not only information about the social system, the substrate for the evolution of the problem, and how it may be currently contributing to improving or maintaining the problem, but also information to better understand the patient's problem.

Family assessment does not necessarily lead to family therapy. If the family assessment reveals a well-functioning family, then reassurance and support can be offered at a time of crisis. A family assessment can be modified depending on the presenting problem. This is similar to varying the elements that one would choose when doing a mental status examination. In the emergency room, a family assessment will initially focus on safety, identification of precipitating factors for relapse or suicidality, and the family's ability to communicate and problem solve. In the inpatient psychiatric unit, these factors can be assessed in more detail, and other possible strengths and weaknesses can be identified. If the family wishes family treatment, then some initial work can be done and further work can be arranged for after discharge. On the consultation service, family assessment may focus on adjustments related to the diagnosis of medical illness, clarification of treatment options, and collaboration in carrying out the treatment plan. This chapter focuses on orienting and assessing families. Chapter 9 will describe the treatment process in greater detail.

An example of a family assessment is shown in the DVD attached to this manual. Appendix 4–1 contains a description of the presenting problems and a written evaluation of this family.

Connecting With the Family

Most beginning therapists, or therapists not used to dealing with families, are anxious when initially sitting with a group of people of whom only one is the identified patient. Psychiatrists in particular may feel especially uneasy in such a situation. Training in the medical model identifies the physician as the source of information, knowledge, control, and the provider of therapy. The families of patients may not see themselves as needing help, may have many questions and/or critical comments about the care of their loved ones, and may appear challenging as a response to their sense of vulnerability in coming into a physician's office. Many families have been blamed, or have felt blamed, for their loved one's illness and may expect to be held accountable once again. Many psychiatrists prefer not to deal with such a potentially uncomfortable situation and relegate family assessments and family interventions to other members of the treatment team. With the proper approach, orientation, and attitude, however, most family meetings can progress smoothly and end with a sense of mutual satisfaction at being able to come to a collaborative understanding of the problem and possible solutions.

The most important step in meeting with a family for the first time is to establish connection with the family. A family needs to feel understood, respected, and validated. They do not want to be blamed for their loved one's problems or judged for their perceived deficiencies. It is the job of the therapist to put families at ease and to make them feel comfortable enough to participate openly and enthusiastically in the assessment process. One effective way of doing this is by orienting the family to the evaluation process.

Orientation

The orientation explains the purpose of the evaluation and establishes goals for the process. It is important to develop a consensus about the agenda when running a meeting. The same process applies to all family meetings; all present must come to an agreement on the purpose of the meeting. This allows everyone to cooperate and work toward the same goals. If family members have different ideas about the agenda, then the assessment process can become difficult and family members may work at cross-purposes.

It is often helpful to start off the meeting with introductions of the participants, including the therapist and any other team members who may be present in the family meeting. The family should be thanked for making the time to come in to meet with the therapist. This recognizes and validates that family members also have important activities and responsibilities in their lives that they have had to put aside for the purpose of helping with the treatment. The process of the meeting is normalized with an explanation that family meetings are a regular part of the assessment and treatment process for all patients. This assures the family that they are not being singled out for blame or that there is anything uniquely problematic about this family.

The family can be further oriented by clarifying why they have come, what they expect will happen, and what they would like to get out of the meeting. These questions will generate useful information and decrease the likelihood of resistance later in the assessment process. The therapist should condense and feed back the family's answers to make sure the family knows that they had been heard and correctly understood. The therapist can then outline his or her expectations from the assessment, explain the rationale for seeing them, and map out the process ahead.

The therapist explains that the goal of the meeting is to provide an opportunity for all family members to identify what they see as problems and to bring up any areas of concern. The therapist lets the family know that this will also be an opportunity for all family members to ask questions of the therapist and/or treatment team in order to give them the same opportunity to address their questions just as the therapist expects the family to address his or her questions. Finally, the family's cooperation in the treatment process is enhanced by letting the family know that the family meeting also provides an opportunity for all family members to have input into the development of a treatment plan.

An opening series of statements is presented as follows:

> "Thank you all for coming in. We like to meet with the families of all of our patients. This is an opportunity for you to let us know how you see what the problems are and to raise any concerns you may have. In order to provide the best treatment, I need to have a clear idea of how you function as a family. I may jump around a bit in order to find out about different aspects of your family life. You will also have a chance to ask any questions that you may have of me. Finally, this will be an opportunity for all of us to put our heads together in order to determine where to go from here. Is that all right with you?"
> **(For an example, see scene 2 in the DVD.)**

Crisis Situations

A comprehensive family assessment may need to be delayed to deal with an immediate crisis. In general, treatment should not start until the family has been evaluated, but there are certain situations in which an intervention may be necessary because of imminent risk to family members. Regardless of how a family functions, a suicidal patient has to be taken care of, violent behavior within a family has to be stopped, and disruptive practices such as substance abuse need to be addressed as soon as possible.

Patients who are imminently suicidal need to be hospitalized or referred to the nearest emergency department. It is clearly not so easy to put a stop to violent behavior in a family or to control substance abuse, as those may be the very problems for which the family is coming to get help. If the family were able to control such behavior, it would be unlikely to be presenting for therapeutic interventions. Nonetheless, if family members continue to be physically abusive toward each other or continue to abuse substances to the point of creating significant symptoms, then treatment cannot take place. Part of the treatment of dangerous and disruptive behaviors consists of putting in place some parameters and structure that allow family members to suspend their usual ways of interacting in a maladaptive way with each other, while they work out longer-term solutions that can help them maintain better control. It is not unreasonable to expect family members to stop their dangerous interactions with each other at least for the duration of the assessment and the initiation of treatment. If they are not able to do even this much, then family interventions may be premature. The victimized family members or the perpetrators may need to be separated and treated individually, oftentimes in a more restrictive environment. This expectation of changing destructive interpersonal behaviors, even in anticipation of the assessment process, may be, in fact, the beginning of treatment.

Even in crisis situations, try to contact another professional who knows the family in order to understand the family context of the presenting problem and plan a crisis intervention.

Composition of Family Meetings

Most family therapists would agree that all members of a family should be seen at least for the initial evaluation. Family can mean anyone who has a significant role in that patient's social situation. This may include in-laws, significant others, friends, and other relatives. It is sometimes helpful to let family members know that they can bring into the family meeting anyone with whom they feel comfortable; this includes anyone who is involved and concerned about the identified patient. It makes sense to try to include an evaluation of all of the people who are likely to play an important role in managing and influencing the patient's problem. In practice, most often, only the immediate family members are likely to come for the family meeting. Bringing in all family members allows the therapist to obtain the full range of family members' views, resulting in a more comprehensive assessment of the situation. It also provides the opportunity for direct observation of family interactions. The therapist cannot come to know the family's way of interacting with each other if significant family members are missing.

Not infrequently, there is one family member who is carrying a disproportionate burden of the family's problems. If appropriately supported, this person can be very helpful in outlining the true nature of the family's issues. This role may fall on a different person in different families. By having all family members come in, there is a greater chance of identifying and including this person in the treatment process. Emphasizing the need for all family members to attend gives a message to the family that everybody is involved in the process and they are all recognized as important people to help bring about change. Other family members may have useful perspectives on the problem and may help identify future resources. It is also easier to include more family members earlier in the treatment process than later. Family members are more likely to mobilize around a crisis and make an effort to put aside their own issues to deal with the crisis, as opposed to after the situation has settled down, at which time people begin once again to become more focused on their own lives.

Young children can contribute a great deal to a family meeting. Parenting skills are assessed by noting if parents bring toys, food, or other supplies to a meeting and if parents can work together successfully to manage the children in the meeting. For example, if one member is talking, then the other member can help by engaging the children in an activity. Asking children such questions as "Who is the boss?" can quickly reveal family structure. Children may be able to answer questions about affect: "How does daddy feel most of the time?" "How does mommy feel?" "What makes you feel sad?" "What makes you feel happy?" Some children may blame themselves for the parent's illness: "If I behaved better, then mommy could come home." Correcting these false beliefs is an important family task. Older children and teenagers can be caregivers for parents or siblings with chronic mental illness or may themselves need care (1). Young people report that they are often ignored by professionals and that they want to be involved in their family member's care and included in decision making. The children may be coping well and may need only support (2). The child's vulnerability depends on age, developmental needs, and the extent and severity of the family member's illness.

After the initial evaluation, during which the greatest number of concerned and interested individuals should participate, decisions can be made about the composition of subsequent meetings. Clearly, if sexual relationships between adults are to be discussed, then the presence of other family members is not appropriate. At different times, due to scheduling problems, it may not be possible for all family members to participate. Having had an opportunity to understand the larger system from the start, however, may help therapists to develop approaches that, at minimum, take into consideration knowledge about the patient's larger social context.

The Evaluation Process

There are many different ways to assess a family and many different kinds of information that can be gathered. It is often confusing for a beginning therapist to try to determine which information is important and how to manage the flow of information in order to make it comprehensible and useful in the formulation that will lead to the treatment. Some family therapists begin with a long history of the family's life, connections, and evolution as a unit. They gather information on families of origin of the members to try to piece together a more comprehensive understanding of the background of the presenting situation. They may develop this through a genogram.

Other therapists are more interested in a here-and-now view of how the family functions and the current problems they are dealing with. They are less concerned about the historical antecedents of the problem and more interested in knowing what the family is struggling with at this time, what they have tried to do about it, and what has or has not worked.

Still other therapists are focused primarily on the process issues in the family session. They address what they observe as the current family interactional pattern and assume that this is representative of the way in which the family struggles with issues outside of the therapy session. By commenting on and clarifying such patterns, they hope to be able to help the family to understand the shape of these patterns without needing to address specific issues in great detail.

All three approaches have merit, and they are not mutually exclusive. The challenge for the therapist is to integrate these three approaches in such a way as to meet the goals of the evaluation without getting unduly sidetracked by peripheral issues or take so long to complete the evaluation that the family loses interest.

We suggest starting the meeting by asking the family to identify what they see as the problems in the family. Each family member is given the opportunity to express his or her concerns without being interrupted by others. The therapist should spend enough time with each family member to ensure that that individual has had an opportunity to outline any problem he or she is concerned about. The challenge for the therapist is to not get sidetracked by beginning to deal with problems before everybody has had an opportunity to present their perspectives. The therapist also has to make sure the problems are not described in such great detail as to leave no time for the exploration of other problems and the concerns of other family members.

Beginning family therapists often get bogged down in detail too early in the list of identified problems. Sometimes they try to treat a situation before all the problems have been identified and delineated, or allow family members to interrupt each other and get into disputes before the problems have been identified, or fail to make sure that each family member has had a chance to identify all concerns.

Individual family members can be kept on track and their comments focused by feeding back to the individual what the therapist heard, to ensure that the correct information has been transmitted and also to let the person know that his or her concerns have been understood. Therefore, he or she does not have to give many examples of the same problem. The therapist should also reassure each family member that his or her concerns will be addressed in due time and that the initial goal is to develop a problem list from all family members. This process is usually not as time-consuming as it may sound. Although each family member can identify many different problems, in reality most family members will agree on a core set of problems, and some of the extraneous problems that are brought up in great detail are likely to be subsumed by more general issues. Even the presenting problems may just be subcomponents of larger, more central family issues. Listening carefully, limiting the amount of detail provided to exemplify each problem, summarizing the therapist's understanding of the problems to reassure family members that they have been heard, and giving everyone the opportunity to speak without interruption should allow for the development of an overview of the range of family members' concerns within a reasonable period of time. The approach will also reassure the family about the therapist's fairness and ability to listen effectively, and it will keep the family from getting caught in their usual style of unproductive problem-solving patterns.

(**For a more comprehensive discussion of the assessment process, see scene 15 in the DVD.**)

Assessment key points

- Include as many family members as possible
- Help family members to describe problems as they experience them
- Evaluate a wide range of family functions
- Consider need for more than one meeting to complete the assessment

---

The Assessment Process

Content of the Assessment

Once the concerns of each family member have been delineated, it is then time to proceed to evaluating the ways in which families function. It is important to know how the family's specific ways of functioning in different spheres of family life contribute to or modify the presenting problem. Assessment of family functioning is analogous to mental status assessment of an individual. It is a way to explore broad dimensions of family life in order to get a better sense of the substrate in which the presented problem exists and to find out which aspects of family interactional patterns can be reinforced to be more helpful and which ones need to be changed.

The assessment is based on family member reports. The therapist confirms the reports by observing the family's behavior in session. At any time, the therapist may clarify contradictions between the stated information and observed behavior and between differing information offered by different family members. The therapist takes care to gather evidence to support his or her hypotheses about family functioning before reflecting them back to the family.

Different models of family functioning have been described, each focused on certain aspects of family life depending on the theoretical orientation and interest of their proponents. The Beavers Systems Model (3), for instance, identifies family competence and family style as two major constructs of family organization. Olson's Circumplex Model of Marital and Family Systems (4) focuses on family cohesion, flexibility, and communications. Moos and Moos

(5) developed a model to assess family interactions that include cohesion, expressiveness, conflict, organization, and control. Expressed emotion, an index of criticalness and overinvolvement by family members with each other, was developed by Brown et al. (6). McCubbin and Thompson (7) stressed the importance of problem-solving ability, adaptability, and cohesion. Miklowitz and Clarkin (8) prioritized problem solving, family organization, and emotional climate. It is clear that there is considerable overlap between these approaches in assessing family interactional and emotional constructs. They are different but overlapping ways of looking at and describing similar phenomena. It is very difficult for a therapist to keep track of these various frameworks while also keeping track of the processes unfolding during a family assessment session. To simplify the task, the therapist needs to pick a set of useful family dimensions to evaluate regularly. This provides a routine structure that ensures a comprehensive and consistent evaluation.

To provide structure to the assessment process similar to the structure provided by a mental status examination checklist, therapists can systematically assess family functioning in the following areas: problem solving, communication, role allocation, affective responsiveness, affective involvement, and behavior control. These dimensions have been taken from the McMaster Model of Family Functioning (9, 10) and are defined below (see "Overall Family Functioning"). The goal of problem solving is to successfully achieve basic developmental and crisis tasks. The goal of communications is to achieve mutual understanding in the family. The goal of role allocation is to achieve satisfactory role integration. The goal of affective responsiveness is to understand the capacity for appropriate emotional reactivity. The goal of affective involvement is to ensure security and autonomy. The goal of behavior control is ensure the maintenance and adaptation of family processes.

Duration of the Assessment

It may take more than one session to do a comprehensive assessment. The number of assessment sessions, of course, will vary depending on the therapist's expertise and the nature of the family's problems. The assessment of the family should not be rushed. It is easy to make assumptions about what is happening and what is important. Without sufficient data to validate or disprove such assumptions, a therapist could easily be treating the wrong problem. In family therapy as in the practice of medicine, there is no substitute for doing a proper diagnostic evaluation before initiating treatment.

In addition to gathering the necessary data for a comprehensive formulation of the problem, a thorough assessment also provides each member of the family the opportunity to offer his or her opinion on family matters, helps family members focus on the appropriate issues, and identifies problems that family members may have not recognized themselves individually. A proper assessment also allows for the identification of family strengths.

If more than one session is needed for a proper assessment, then this needs to be discussed with the family. It is important to summarize the findings of the assessment to date and let the family know that more information is needed before a decision can be made regarding the diagnosis and treatment of the problem. The assessment sessions, if there is more than one, should not be spaced more than a week apart, to avoid dragging the process out.

Although a comprehensive assessment is necessary, it is important to complete it as efficiently as possible. Families may not return for subsequent sessions if they feel much information is being gathered from them without their receiving any feedback as to what it means. Families need to have feedback along the way, outlining the therapist's understanding of the problems and the direction that the assessment process is heading, to keep them engaged.

Gathering Identifying Data

Before evaluating particular dimensions of family functioning, it is necessary to obtain information about family members' names, ages, relationships within the family, and living arrangements. It is also helpful to ascertain the current phase of the family life cycle to anticipate the kinds of problems and issues that the family may be struggling with in addition to the presenting problem.

Once the presenting problems are clearly delineated by the various family members, and once the therapist has summarized his or her understanding of these problems with consensus of all participants that the problems are understood and agreed upon, the therapist moves on to assess the dimensions of family functioning. The goal of this stage of the assessment is to complete the assessment by checking out areas of family functioning that may not have been presented during the delineation of the identified problems. Just as a patient with depression may not necessarily volunteer that he or she has auditory hallucinations or could hurt him- or herself for being "a bad person," a family may not identify problems in the family without being asked to elaborate on them. The therapist asks a series of focused questions about the dimensions of family functioning as a way of scanning the family's ability to deal with each other and the pressures that they are facing. This broader understanding of the family's functioning in various domains of family life is an important part of the development of an appropriate treatment plan.

Dimensions of family functioning

- Problem solving
- Communication
- Roles
- Affective responsiveness
- Affective involvement
- Behavior control

Overall Family Functioning

The therapist orients the family to this stage of exploration by a comment such as, "Now we'd like to switch to get a general idea of how you operate as a family. I am going to ask you a series of questions about different aspects of your family life. Is that all right?" As the examination of each dimension of family functioning progresses, the therapist should provide feedback on his or her understanding of the assets and shortcomings for each particular area.

Problem solving.   Problem solving refers to a family's ability to resolve problems to a level that maintains effective family functioning. A family problem is an issue that threatens the integrity and functional capacity of the family and that the family has difficulty solving. Family problems are divided into two types: instrumental and affective. Instrumental problems refer to problems of everyday life, such as managing money and obtaining food, clothing, and housing. Affective problems concern issues of emotion or feeling, such as anger or depression. Families whose functioning is disrupted by instrumental problems rarely deal effectively with affective problems. Families who have problems with affective issues, however, may be able to adequately address instrumental problems.

Stages of effective problem solving include identifying the problem, communicating about it with an appropriate person or persons, developing alternatives, deciding on an alternative, and acting on that decision. Finally, the problem-solving process is monitored and its effectiveness is evaluated at its conclusion.

Questions about problem-solving skills of the family may be general, or, if the family has trouble abstracting about their problem-solving procedures, family members can be asked to think of family problems that have come up within the last few weeks to use as an example. The following questions may be helpful in exploring the family's effectiveness in managing problems:

- Who first notices problems?
- What did you do after you noticed the problem?
- Did you discuss it with anybody?
- What did you decide to do about the problem?
- Did you think of any alternatives?
- Did you discuss how you dealt with the problem once you had taken care of it?
- How do you handle practical problems?
- How do you handle problems that involve emotions?

(For an example, see scene 7 in the DVD.)

Communication.   Communication refers to the verbal exchange of information within a family. Nonverbal communication is very important as well, but it is more difficult to quantify and monitor. Communication can also be thought of as instrumental or affective. Families can have marked difficulties with the affective component of communication but can function very well in the instrumental area. Communication can also be thought of as clear versus masked. Masked communication tends to be camouflaged, muddied, or vague. Communication can also be direct or indirect. Indirect communication tends to get deflected from the intended target to someone else. Families with poor functioning tend to have unclear and/or indirect forms of communication. Questions assessing the communication dimension can be as follows:

- Do people in this family talk with one another?
- Can you talk about practical things with each other?
- Can you talk about emotional issues with each other?
- Do you feel that you can talk things through with others in the family, or do you have to be guarded about what you say?
- Can you tell things to each other directly, or do you have to use someone else to let others know how you feel and think?

   (For an example, see scene 6 in the DVD.)

Role allocation.   Roles are the repetitive patterns of behavior by which family members fulfill family functions. Family functions include the provision of resources, nurturance and support, sexual gratification, personal development, and maintenance and management of the family system, the last including decision making, boundaries and membership functions, and household finances and management.

   Questions to explore the role dimension of families include the following:

- How do you divide responsibilities?
- Who works and for how many hours?
- Who handles the money?
- Who buys the groceries and prepares the meals?
- Who does the housework?
- Who looks after the home and cars?
- Who oversees what happens with the children's education?
- Who gets involved with the schools?
- Who is involved in major decisions?
- Who has the final say?
- How do you decide who does what job?
- Do you feel that some people have too many jobs?
- Do any of you feel overburdened by your jobs?
- Are the responsibilities fairly shared between family members? If not, how would you like to see it done differently?

   (For an example, see scene 10 in the DVD.)

Affective responsiveness.   Affective responsiveness evaluates whether family members are able to respond to the full spectrum of feelings experienced in emotional life and whether the emotion experienced is consistent or appropriate with the stimulus, situation, or context. This dimension assesses an individual's capacity to a greater extent than do the other family dimensions. Affective responsiveness is different from affective communication in that responsiveness refers to the person's capacity to experience a particular affect. Affective communication refers to how family members transmit to each other emotions they are experiencing. The affective responsiveness dimension attempts to evaluate the capacity of individual family members to experience affect in order to determine whether family members tend to be overcome with feelings or are not sufficiently capable of experiencing them. There are two broad types of affect that can be assessed. *Welfare emotions* consist of affection, warmth, tenderness, support, love, consolation, happiness, and joy. *Emergency emotions* encompass fear, anger, sadness, disappointment, and depression.

It is useful to know if some of the family difficulties may be a function of particular individuals' under- or overresponsiveness to affective stimuli. The following questions elicit information regarding emotional responses:

- Are you a family that responds to situations with a lot of feeling?
- Do any of you feel that you are a family who underresponds in terms of emotions?
- Which kinds of emotions do you think you overrespond or underrespond to?
- Do others sense that you do not experience feelings that you should feel or that you think others do?
- Are there any feelings that you experience more intensely than you think is reasonable given the situation?
  (For an example, see scene 9 in the DVD.)

Affective involvement.   Affective involvement refers to the extent to which the family shows interest in and values the activities of individual family members. Families can lack involvement with each other and not show any interest in each other. They coexist in the same space without much connection. Some family members are narcissistically involved. Here, the investment in others is only in terms of what that individual can get out of it without concern for the other. With empathic involvement, family members demonstrate true concern for the interests of others in the family, even though these concerns may be peripheral to their own interests. Overinvolvement and symbiotic involvement tend to be overintrusive and overprotective, sometimes to the point that boundaries between family members are blurred significantly. Questions that can help explore aspects of affective involvement include the following:

- Who cares about what is important to you?
- Do you think other family members are interested in you?
- Do they ever show too much interest?
- Do you feel that they are truly interested in you because it is important to you or only because they think they should be?
- Do you feel that other members of the family go their own way and do not care or notice what happens to you?

(For an example, see scene 8 in the DVD.)

Behavior control.   The behavior control dimension evaluates the ways in which a family establishes rules about acceptable behavior relating to physically dangerous situations, situations involving meeting and expressing psychobiological needs and drives, and situations involving socializing behavior between family members and people outside the family. This dimension concerns parental discipline toward children as well as standards and expectations of behavior that adults set for each other. There are a variety of styles of behavior control, including rigid behavior control, flexible behavior control, laissez-faire behavior control (where there are no standards or direction), and chaotic behavior control (where standards shift in a random and unpredictable fashion between rigid, flexible, and laissez-faire and family members do not know which standards apply at any one time).

The following questions can be used to explore the behavior control dimension of family functioning:

- Do you have rules in your family about how to handle different situations?
- How do you handle dangerous situations?
- Do you have rules for table manners and for bedtime?
- Do you allow hitting or yelling at each other?
- Do you know what is expected of you in terms of behavior with people outside the family?

- Do you have rules about drinking? Driving too fast? Letting people know where you are when you are away from home?
- Are the rules clear?
- Are the rules the same for everybody?
- Can you discuss the rules to change them?
- Do you always know what the family expect?
- Do you know what they expect if the rules are broken?

(**For an example, see scene 11 in the DVD.**)

Dysfunctional Transactional Patterns

Throughout the assessment stage, the therapist identifies potentially dysfunctional transactional patterns. These patterns are repetitive interactional processes that prevent effective resolution of ongoing interpersonal problems. It is not necessary to immediately label and deal with dysfunctional transactional patterns early in the assessment stage, particularly if this distracts from completing a thorough assessment. It is useful to take mental note of the pattern and proceed with the rest of the assessment. If the pattern does recur, it is often in association with the presenting problem.

During the later stages of the assessment process, the therapist may recognize a consistent dysfunctional transactional pattern that seems associated with problems in several dimensions. The therapist may label the process directly at this point to see if the family agrees with the observation and shows interest in doing something about it.

A transactional pattern that is disruptive may need to be identified early to allow for the assessment to continue without being derailed. However, the therapist must not be sidetracked with treatment too early in the assessment process before a full understanding of the family has been achieved. Dysfunctional transactional patterns may also be a family's way of deflecting attention away from more significant problems by creating conflicts that feel less threatening to them.

(**For an example, see scene 5 in the DVD.**)

Tools for Family Assessment

A variety of instruments exist to evaluate families systematically. Instruments allow for numerical quantification of family functioning, including tracking of change over time, comparison with other families, and the opportunity for quantitative and qualitative research. Family evaluation tools are either objective or subjective.

Subjective family rating scales are self-report paper-and-pencil or computer touch-screen instruments filled out by family members. These instruments elicit individual family members' views of their own family's functioning. One benefit of subjective family instruments is cost-effectiveness. Because they are self-report instruments, family members can fill them out at their leisure, and the assessment does not require trained interviewer time. Family members usually fill out the questionnaires in less than 30 minutes. They do not require manuals to complete, can be easily transported to a variety of settings, and can be compared over time. A potential problem in understanding subjective perspectives of family functioning is how to integrate the views of different family members, especially if they are different from each other. A variety of approaches have been developed to try to merge individual family members' perspectives on their family's functioning. One way is to average individual scores and arrive at an overall family score. Another way is to look at differences in the perception of various family members. Scores on these instruments can be used to track changes in families over time, particularly as it relates to ongoing treatment.

The disadvantage of self-report instruments is that they are restricted to an internal perspective of family functioning and may not reflect the way a family appears to function to an outside observer. Not all family assessment instruments are reliable or have been validated. Different scales emphasize different aspects of family functioning or measure the same concept differently, depending on the model from which they are derived.

Externally rated instruments of family functioning administered by trained interviewers provide an objective view of the family's functioning. These structured or semistructured interview instruments are independent of the family's tendency to want to see themselves in a particular way. They provide more reliable assessments for comparisons between different families and comparison with established population norms. A disadvantage of externally rated family assessment instruments is their relative expense; interviewers have to be trained to rate families reliably, and these instruments take a longer time to administer.

Self-report instruments of family functioning

- Dyadic Adjustment Scale
- Self-Report Family Inventory
- Family Environment Scale
- Family Adaptability and Cohesion Evaluation Scales III
- Family Assessment Device

There is no absolute advantage to either an external or an internal perspective on family functioning. Both perspectives are important, and each may be relatively more useful to answer different kinds of questions. A family's view of itself, for instance, may be just as important as an external observer's evaluation of the family, even if the two views are different. A discrepancy between an outside evaluator and family members' perception of their family's functioning and differences between individual family members' views of their own family's functioning may provide particularly useful clinical information about that family's problems over and above the specific results of either form of assessment. The information from both kinds of assessments can be complementary to each other. Since neither is necessarily more or less accurate, which one is used will depend on the questions being asked and the time and resources available to undertake the evaluation.

In the following sections we list a number of commonly used scales. The list is not comprehensive.

Externally rated instruments of family functioning

- Global Assessment of Relational Functioning
- Beavers Interactional Styles Scale
- Camberwell Family Interview
- McMaster Clinical Rating Scale

Self-Report Instruments

Brief, useful self-report measures of marital adjustment/satisfaction and family functioning are available for the practicing clinician. Family members can fill these out in the waiting room or at home, before the first session, and during the course of treatment as a way of monitoring progress. The following are examples of commonly used instruments.

- *Dyadic Adjustment Scale* (11): measures satisfaction, cohesion, consensus, and affectional expression in couples.
- *Self-Report Family Inventory* (12): assesses conflict resolution, styles of relating, intergenerational boundaries, and family competence.
- *Family Environment Scale* (5): assesses relationship (cohesion, expressiveness, conflict), personal growth (independence, achievement, morality/religion), and system maintenance (organization, control).
- *Family Adaptability and Cohesion Evaluation Scales III* (4): measures adaptability (rules, power structure, roles) and cohesion (emotional bonding, autonomy, boundaries).
- *Family Assessment Device* (13): assesses the dimensions of the McMaster Model of Family Functioning—problem solving, communication, role allocation, affective responsiveness, affective involvement, behavior control, and general functioning.

Externally Rated Family Assessment Instruments

Observer-rated couples and family interaction instruments provide a more objective perspective of a family's way of dealing with each other and the world around them. The following are some of the commonly used instruments.

Global Assessment of Relational Functioning

The Global Assessment of Relational Functioning (GARF) scale (Table 4–1) is similar to the individual focused Global Assessment of Functioning (GAF) (14) but focuses instead on relational adjustment and also on the quality of the family environment. The GARF measures relational functioning in the same way that the GAF measures general individual functioning, on a scale of 1 to 99. The GARF is a composite of the three most researched family assessment tools: the Beavers Systems Model, the Olsen Circumplex Model, and the McMaster Model. Three areas are assessed: interactional problem solving, organization, and emotional climate. The GARF is included in Appendix B of DSM-IV-TR (American Psychiatric Association 2000) as a set of criteria needing further study (15). The GARF allows the clinician to document relational functioning on a scale that includes healthy family functioning and is an important step toward the recognition of family strengths as important components of a patient's presentation.

Beavers Interactional Styles Scale

The Beavers Interactional Styles Scale (12) evaluates a family's competence and style. It also assesses power, parental coalitions, clarity of expression, conflict, negotiation, responsibility, and empathy.

Camberwell Family Interview

The Camberwell Family Interview (16) measures expressed emotion, the amount of criticism expressed by family members about each other, and emotional overinvolvement (the extent to which family members are involved in each other's lives and concerns).

McMaster Clinical Rating Scale

The McMaster Clinical Rating Scale (17) is an interviewer assessment (with the aid of the McMaster Structured Interview of Family Functioning if desired) of a family's communications, problem solving, affective involvement, affective responsiveness, roles, behavior control, and general functioning.

DSM-IV Relational Diagnoses

Relational problems are described in DSM-IV-TR in a section titled "Other Conditions That May Be a Focus of Clinical Attention." Five relational problems are described as V codes. According to DSM-IV-TR (15):

> These problems may exacerbate or complicate the management of a mental disorder or general medical condition in one or more members, may be a result of a mental illness, or a general medical condition, may be independent of other conditions that are present or can occur in the absence of other conditions. When these problems are the principal focus of clinical attention, they should be listed on Axis I. Otherwise, they may be listed on Axis IV. (pp. 736–737).

Table 4–1.   The Global Assessment of Relational Functioning (GARF) Scale

Rating

81–99   Family functioning is satisfactory.

61–80   Family functioning is somewhat unsatisfactory.

41–60   Family has occasional time of satisfactory functioning, but unsatisfactory relationships predominate.

21–40   Family is obviously and seriously dysfunctional.

1–20   Family is too dysfunctional to retain continuity, contact, and attachment.

GARF Subscales

Interactional/Problem solving

Skills in negotiating goals, rules, and routines; adaptability to stress, communication skills; ability to resolve conflict.

81–100   Agreed-on patterns or routines exist that help meet the usual needs of each family/couple member; there is flexibility for change in response to unusual demands or events; and occasional conflicts and stressful transitions are resolved through problem-solving communication and negotiation.

61–80   Daily routines are present, but there is some pain and difficulty in responding to the unusual. Some conflicts remain unresolved but do not disrupt family functioning.

41–60   Communication is frequently inhibited by unresolved conflicts that often interfere with daily routines; there is significant difficulty in adapting to family stress and transitional change.

21–40   Family/couple routines do not meet the needs of members; they are grimly adhered to or blithely ignored. Life cycle changes, such as departures or entries into the relational unit, generate painful conflict and obviously frustrating failures of problem solving.

Organization

Maintenance of interpersonal roles and subsystem boundaries; hierarchical functioning; coalitions and distribution of power, control, and responsibility.

81–100   There is a shared understanding and agreement about roles and appropriate tasks, decision making is established for each functional area, and there is recognition of the unique characteristics and merit of each subsystem (e.g., parents/spouses, siblings, and individuals).

Table 4–1. The Global Assessment of Relational Functioning (GARF) Scale *(continued)*

61–80 Decision making is usually competent, but efforts at control of one another quite often are greater than necessary or are ineffective. Individuals and relationships are clearly demarcated but sometimes a specific subsystem is depreciated or scapegoated.

41–60 Decision making is only intermittently competent and effective; either excessive rigidity or significant lack of structure is evident at these times. Individual needs are quite often submerged by a partner or coalition.

21–40 Decision making is tyrannical or quite ineffective. The unique characteristics of individuals are unappreciated or ignored by either rigid or confusingly fluid coalitions.

1–20 Family/couple members are not organized in such a way that personal or generational responsibilities are recognized. Boundaries of relational unit as a whole and subsystems cannot be identified or agreed on. Family members are physically endangered or injured or sexually attacked.

Emotional climate

Tone and range of feelings; quality of caring, empathy, involvement, and attachment/ commitment; sharing of values; mutual affective responsiveness, respect, and regard; quality of sexual functioning.

81–100 Situationally appropriate, optimistic atmosphere in family; a wide range of feelings is freely expressed and managed within family; and a general atmosphere of warmth, caring, and sharing of values among all family members. Sexual relations of adult members are satisfactory.

61–80 A range of feeling is expressed, but emotional blocking or tension is evident. Warmth and caring are present but marred by irritability and frustrations. Sexual activity of adult members may be problematic.

41–60 Pain or ineffective anger or emotional deadness interferes with family enjoyment. Although there is some warmth and support for members, it is usually unequally distributed. Troublesome sexual difficulties between adults are often present.

21–40 There are infrequent periods of enjoyment of life together; frequent distancing or open hostility reflects significant conflicts that remain unresolved. Sexual dysfunction among adult members is commonplace.

1–20 Despair and cynicism are pervasive; there is little attention to the emotional needs of others; there is almost no sense of attachment, commitment, or concern about one another's welfare.

Source. Adapted from American Psychiatric Association: *Diagnostic and Statistical Manual of Mental Disorders*, 4th Edition, Text Revision. Washington, DC, American Psychiatric Association, 2000. Copyright 2000, American Psychiatric Association. Used with permission.

V codes for relational problems

- V61.9   Relational problem related to a mental disorder or general medical condition
- V61.10   Partner relational problem
- V61.20   Parent-child relational problem
- V61.8   Sibling relational problem
- V62.81   Relational problem not otherwise specified

Problems related to abuse or neglect are included in this section under V61.21. These include physical abuse of child, sexual abuse of child, neglect of child, physical abuse of adult, and sexual abuse of adult.

Conclusion

A systematic assessment of the family is central to understanding the pertinent issues in a family and its potential role in shaping a patient's presenting problem. This understanding contributes to a comprehensive biopsychosocial formulation (Chapter 6) leading to a treatment plan that is likely to address most of the variables that may need and could benefit from clinical interventions. To be able to perform a systematic family assessment, the therapist would find it useful to have a consistent, broadly based, and structured assessment template. Such a template ensures that a wide range of family dimensions is assessed and helps the therapist stay on track. In addition to the standard clinical interview, there are also subjective and objective assessment instruments to help in the evaluation process. These instruments complement the clinical evaluation and can track changes over time systematically. A good family assessment is therapeutic in and of itself even if the decision is made that no further family intervention is indicated.

References

1. Fudge E, Falkov A, Kowalenko N, et al: Parenting is a mental health issue. Australas Psychiatry 12:166, 2004

2. Falcov A, Lindsey C: Patients as parents: addressing the needs including the safety of children where parents have mental illness, in Council Report CR 105. London, Royal College of Psychiatrists, 2002

3. Beavers WR, Hampson RB: Measuring family competence: the Beavers systems model, in Normal Family Processes: Growing Diversity and Complexity, 3rd Edition. Edited by Walsh F. New York, Guilford, 2003, pp 549–580

4. Olson DH, Russell CS, Sprenkle DH: Circumplex Model: Systemic Assessment and Treatment of Families. New York, Haworth, 1989

5. Moos R, Moos B: Family Environment Scale Manual. Palo Alto, CA, Consulting Psychologists Press, 1981

6. Brown G, Monck E, Carstairs G: Influence of family life on the course of schizophrenic illness. Br J Prev Soc Med 68:55–68, 1962

7. McCubbin HI, Thompson AI: Family hardiness index, in Family Assessment Inventories for Research and Practice. Madison, University of Wisconsin, 1987, pp 124–130

8. Miklowitz DJ, Clarkin JF: Diagnosis of family relational disorders, in Textbook of Family and Couples Therapy. Edited by Sholevar GP, Schwoeri LD. Washington, DC, American Psychiatric Publishing, 2003, pp 341–366

9. Epstein NB, Keitner GI, Bishop DS, et al: Combined use of pharmacological and family therapy, in Affective Disorders and the Family. Edited by Clarkin JF, Hass G, Glick I. New York, Guilford, 1988, pp 153–172

10. Ryan CE, Epstein N, Keitner GI, et al: Evaluating and Treating Families: The McMaster Approach. New York, Routledge Taylor & Francis Group, 2005

11. Spanier GB: Measuring dyadic adjustment: new scales for assessing the quality of marriage and similar dyads. J Marriage Fam 38:15–28, 1976

12. Beavers R, Hampson RB: Successful Families: Assessment and Intervention. New York, WW Norton, 1990

13. Epstein NB, Baldwin LM, Bishop DS: The McMaster family assessment device. J Marital Fam Ther 9:203–208, 1983

14. Rosen KH, McCollum EE, Middletown K, et al: Interrater reliability and validity of the Global Assessment of Relational Functioning (GARF) scale in a clinical setting: a preliminary study. Am J Fam Ther 25:357–360, 1997

15. American Psychiatric Association Work Group on Depressive Disorders: Practice guidelines for the treatment of patients with depressive disorder (revision). Am J Psychiatry 157 (suppl), 2000

16. Brown GW, Rutter M: The measurement of family activities and relationships: a methodological study. Hum Relat 19:241–263, 1966

17. Miller IW, Kabacoff RI, Epstein NB, et al: The development of a clinical rating scale for the McMaster Model of Family Functioning. Fam Process 33:53–69, 1994

Appendix 4–1. Case Example

Family Assessment and Treatment Contracting

The purpose of the DVD is to show how to engage a family, perform a comprehensive evaluation of the family within a reasonable time frame, and establish a treatment plan. In viewing the DVD, therapists will find it is more helpful to focus on the process of family assessment rather than the particulars of the patient's illness. The assessment includes an evaluation of the relationship between and among family members as they participate in the assessment. In addition to answers to the specific questions, pay attention to the flow of the assessment, sequence of questions, involvement of the family in the process, and identification of transactional patterns. The challenge for the therapist is to obtain sufficient information to be able to complete a comprehensive evaluation of the family and the presenting problems while at the same time being sensitive to the individual needs and concerns of all family members. The therapist should not be mechanical and rigid in assessing the various dimensions of family functioning but also not be sidetracked in an attempt to deal with specific family concerns until the evaluation has been completed.

This family consists of the mother, who has dysthymia with superimposed episodes of major depression; the father; a daughter who has returned to live at home after completing college; and a son who lives away from home in another state. The family presents for treatment with concerns about family dissension and frustration resulting from the mother's depression, her negativity, a perceived inability to be satisfied, and the father and daughter's confusion as to how to be able to help her when she is depressed. The mother has been in treatment for depression for many years (psychotherapy and pharmacotherapy) but feels that the treatments have not been helpful. She continues to feel chronically "low" and has depressive episodes lasting 4–6 weeks one to two times per year. She works as a social worker, the father as a teacher, and the daughter as a waitress. The mother has a strong family history of depression. There are no other significant illnesses in any of the other family members.

Assessment. The family presented for help in dealing with the mother's depression and the estrangement that they were increasingly feeling from each other. The problems in the family had been getting progressively worse since the children left home for college. They have become exacerbated by the recent return of the daughter after graduation. Their son left home to work in another area of the country 2 years previously. The mother feels misunderstood and unsupported by her husband and upset with her daughter for not moving on with her life independently. The father feels frustrated by his wife's negativism, unavailability to him, and lack of intimacy. The daughter feels that her mother is never satisfied with her performance and nags her excessively about having returned home.

Problem solving: Their problem-solving skills are fair. They can identify problems and delegate responsibility for taking care of them to the appropriate person. The mother usually identifies problems and delegates resolution of the problems to the father. Difficulties arise when they disagree about solutions to problems, as they do not have an effective way of communicating about and resolving differences of opinion. They have significant difficulties in resolving affective problems, the main reason for seeking treatment. The father feels frustrated at not being able to "fix" his wife's depression and has withdrawn from her as a way of dealing with his sense of helplessness.

Communication: The family has difficulties in talking with each other about both instrumental and affective issues. They tend not to listen to each other, especially around issues related to the mother's mood. The father is hesitant to talk with his wife about the frustration he feels out of fear of causing her symptoms to worsen. The father and daughter can talk about daily issues but not about their concerns about the mother's depression. Communications are masked and indirect. The father acts as a messenger between his wife and daughter. Family members disagree about many things and do not have a good way of resolving differences. They spend very little time talking with each other. Many issues remained unresolved, as they are not able to talk with each other without getting into arguments. They feel as if they are "walking on eggshells."

Role allocation: The family has a traditional way of allocating roles. The mother takes care of household responsibilities (cooking, cleaning, shopping, laundry) and the father looks after bills, repairs, and car maintenance. They feel satisfied with the distribution of responsibilities. They are not good at providing nurturance and support for each other concerning their professional and personal developmental needs. The daughter has very few responsibilities and is felt to be an additional burden at this time. The couple report some stresses with their families of origin. Lack of sexual intimacy is a serious concern.

Affective responsiveness: The father and daughter are able to experience a full range of emotions appropriately. They both feel sad and angry about the mother's inability to manage her depression. The mother is able to experience pleasure at times. She is burdened with excessive feelings of sadness. She is angry at her husband for not meeting her emotional needs.

Affective involvement: The mother and father feel isolated and unsupported by the other. They cannot turn to each other. The father feels that his wife is concerned about him, whereas the wife feels that her husband is unavailable to meet her emotional needs. The father cares about his wife's welfare and is committed to the relationship. He finds it difficult to get close to her due to her fluctuating mood and has retreated into his own space. The wife is more ambivalent about her connection and commitment to her husband and is contemplating a separation. The couple had shared common interests in the past but has grown apart over the years and spends very little enjoyable time together now. The mother is concerned that her daughter is assuming too much of a caretaking role with her to compensate for her husband's emotional absence. The daughter feels that both parents are concerned about her and are available to her. Overall the family members are disconnected from each other. Feeling misunderstood and unsupported, they retreat into their own space, sharing a house but not their lives.

Behavior control: There is clear understanding about family rules and expectations. There are no problems with inconsistent, dangerous, or disruptive behaviors. They are respectful of each other.

Transactional patterns. The wife's inability to talk about her depression and the husband's frustration at not being able to "fix" it has led them to withdraw from each other and to not be able to discuss any emotionally charged issue. She is critical, so he withdraws; she feels abandoned, sad, and angry, which leads him to pull back further. The family members often misinterpret each other and feel that they are walking on eggshells much of the time. The son has left the home, in part, to get away from this pressure. The daughter has come home, in part, to meet her mother's emotional needs. This has resulted in the mother feeling guilty, the father not having to deal with his withdrawal, and the daughter putting her own life on hold. They argue and fight with each other as a way to connect.

Formulation. The mother has a biological vulnerability to depression as evidenced by a strong family history of depression and a chronic pattern of "double" depression. She has tried both individual psychotherapy and pharmacotherapy with little benefit. Over the years the mother and father have drifted apart secondary to ongoing episodes of depression and an inability to discuss concerns and frustrations with each other. The presence of their children gave them a common purpose. This was lost when the children left home, leading to a worsening of her depression and the couple's relationship. The daughter has returned home partly to help provide emotional support for her mother. The mother, however, feels guilty and ashamed that her daughter senses this need, and the mother expresses this by being critical and becoming more depressed. She is angry at her husband for not being available to her. The husband has withdrawn because he feels hurt, frustrated, and helpless. The couple is devoid of intimacy. There is recognition that the family's way of dealing with each other has become dysfunctional for all family members and that the wife's depression may not be responding to pharmacotherapy or individual therapy partly because the family problems have not been addressed.

Contracting. The family is given the option of continuing their situation as it is, trying to change it themselves, trying other forms of treatment, or engaging in family therapy. They choose to participate in family therapy.

As indices of their commitment to improve ways of connecting and interacting with each other, they agree to the following first steps:

Wife's requests:

- The husband to be at the dinner table at an agreed-upon time.
- The husband and wife to spend one half day of each weekend doing something together.

Husband's requests:

- At dinner, the wife will talk about their day rather than focus on problems with their children or her depressed mood.
- The wife will greet him when he comes home and ask about how his day went.

Parents' requests of daughter:

- Clean her room or close the door.
- Do her own laundry.

Daughter's request of parents:

- Take care of each other's needs better so that she does not feel the need to provide for them what they are not getting from each other.

5

Site-Specific Family Assessment

- If the clinical situation precludes completion of a full family assessment, then a focused family assessment can evaluate a family's ability to communicate, solve problems, allocate roles, and provide safety for its members.
- Emergency situations require intervention before a comprehensive family assessment is completed.
- At a minimum, an attempt should be made to obtain family members' perspectives on the patient's presenting problems.

Specific clinical settings require modification of the family assessment. A comprehensive family assessment should be deferred in emergency situations, such as the need for immediate treatment of a psychotic, suicidal, violent, or intoxicated patient or to manage the fear of violence or abuse. A family assessment may also need to be abbreviated because of time constraints. In the emergency room or on a medical floor, the patient may not be able to tolerate a full family assessment. In these cases, it is wise to pick the most pertinent area for assessment and defer further family assessment to a follow-up meeting. The family assessment is carried out in the same way as a mental status examination; that is, the assessment is as complete as the clinical situation and time allow and covers the key areas. In this chapter, the process is described using the same principles in each case: orientation, assessment, formulation, and discussion of treatment plan.

Orientation

Just as it is important to develop a consensus about the agenda when running any meeting, the same thing applies to a family meeting. All present must agree on the purpose of the meeting. This allows everyone to cooperate and work toward the same goals. If family members have different ideas about the agenda, then the assessment process can become difficult and family members may talk at cross-purposes. The content of the orientation depends on the site of the evaluation. The complexity of the orientation depends on the urgency of the situation. A brief agreement is sufficient for an emergency situation, whereas a full commitment and understanding of the assessment process and how it differs from treatment is needed for a more complete outpatient assessment.

Assessment

A family assessment usually means an assessment of the family with whom the patient lives but can refer to extended family members and members of a group home, a mental health center case manager, or even involved neighbors and friends. A conference call may be needed if a significant family member is not able to attend the meeting. The assessment should proceed using the framework and guidelines outlined in Chapter 4. It is important to keep as broad a perspective as the situation permits. Focusing too narrowly on details of the presenting problem or getting sidetracked to deal prematurely with peripheral issues before developing an understanding of the broader context of the problem may lead to missing more central conflicts. **Ways to avoid being sidetracked are illustrated in the assessment scenes (1 through 14) of the DVD and discussed in scene 15.** Patients and families may be ambivalent about or afraid of addressing central issues and may instead present less threatening concerns. A more systematic review of family functioning and the broader social context of the presenting problems reduce the likelihood of missing key issues.

If time is limited and the setting does not allow a full assessment to be completed, what aspects of the assessment should be chosen? This is a clinical decision, based on what facts are known about the case. For example, patients, especially adolescents, often present when the family is having difficulties transitioning to the next developmental stage. For adolescents, questions about problem solving and behavioral control are pertinent. When a patient presents with suicidality, it is important to assess how well the family can problem solve and communicate about affective issues. It is worth spending a few minutes before the assessment to consider family developmental issues pertinent to the case and issues that might be important for follow-up planning. In this way, time can be spent wisely. However, often the key issues do not emerge until the assessment is under way.

Formulation

A complete case formulation summarizes the biological, psychological, and social aspects of the problem. There are many advantages to a biopsychosocial formulation. First, it ensures that an attempt is made to explore the likely multivariate nature of the presenting problems. Focusing on only one dimension of a problem is likely to lead to an incomplete understanding and a limited approach to its resolution. Second, a broad formulation engages the family in an exploration of all pertinent factors, framing the family as an important resource and empowering the family to participate in problem solving. Finally, a comprehensive formulation sets realistic expectations about which interventions may or may not be helpful with different aspects of the problem. A complete formulation is often not possible in a crisis situation. In such situations, the therapist needs to be as comprehensive as is feasible.

The formulation is presented to the family for confirmation and to clarify points of disagreement. The psychiatrist emphasizes that the family agrees that a problem exists, not necessarily that they agree on causes or solutions. The psychiatrist works with the patient and family to reach an understanding of the problem. (**Watch how the psychiatrist seeks continued agreement from the family throughout the assessment process on the DVD, especially in scenes 3 and 4, where the presenting problems are assessed. This checking and rechecking for consensus is further discussed in scene 13.**)

When there is disagreement about the existence of specific problems, then the psychiatrist must clarify each family member's position. For example, the patient with substance abuse/dependence may not agree with the formulation that is focused on his or her need for abstinence. The psychiatrist can facilitate a discussion with family members regarding what they are willing to tolerate if the patient continues to abuse substances. The family benefits by discussing limit setting, for example, money and access to resources. Involving the family even if the patient does not stop using substances can benefit the patient (1). A formulation that includes a discussion of prodromal signs and symptoms and an agreement that these signs and symptoms are the indication to make an immediate appointment can prevent relapse.

Treatment Planning

The first step is to engage the family, to make sure that they feel heard and understood and that they have a clear idea of what can or cannot be done to address the problem.

The treatment of the patient and family may not include formal family therapy or in fact any type of family work. If family treatment is part of the treatment plan, a decision needs to be made as to what level of family involvement is appropriate, for example, supportive, psychoeducational, or in-depth family therapy that focuses on structural or affective change. The specific treatment of patients and their families is described in Chapters 8, 9, and 11.

Case Examples

Family Assessment in the Emergency Room

Mr. and Mrs. S bring their 17-year-old son, Jeffrey, to the emergency room. He has been suspended from school after alcohol and marijuana were found in his backpack. This is the second time he has been caught with alcohol at school. The family reports that Jeffrey has been behaving aggressively at home; he has been withdrawn and, when confronted, becomes angry and belligerent. The parents want him assessed so that he can return to school. This information has been obtained by telephone from the school nurse who made the referral to the emergency room. In the waiting area, Jeffrey is slumped down in his chair, his baseball cap covering his face; he appears to be asleep. The parents look concerned and angry, and they communicate little with each other. The father is focused on some papers in his lap, while the mother tries to get Jeffrey and his younger brother, Ryan, to sit up in their chairs and talk to her. Ryan is playing a game on his cell phone and prefers to lie on the floor.

Situational modifications to a comprehensive assessment of the family

- Emergency situations
- Time constraints
- Logistic obstacles
- Outpatient clinic

Orientation: Dr. J invites the patient and his family into an assessment room. After introductions, she begins: "I understand that you are all here because you are concerned about Jeffrey. I have spoken with the school nurse who has filled me in a little. What I would like to do is spend some time with the whole family first, getting everyone's input, and then I would like to talk privately with Jeffrey. Is that all right with everyone?" Mr. and Mrs. S and Ryan agree. Jeffrey ignores Dr. J. "Jeffrey, it is important that I hear from you. Is it okay that we all talk together for a while and then we talk privately?" Jeffrey grudgingly agrees, nodding his head and making brief eye contact. It is important to engage all family members as soon as possible. Dr. J's redoubled efforts toward Jeffrey reassure him that his input is important. This brief orientation suffices for the emergency room.

Assessment: Dr. J begins with some questions to assess problem solving. "Who first noticed that Jeffrey was having a problem?" The mother answers in a rambling way beginning with Jeffrey's first day in kindergarten. Although this information is not directly relevant for an emergency room assessment, Dr. J listens for a few minutes and watches the reaction of other family members. The father and the boys pay no attention to the mother. Jeffrey continues to examine his shoes. "Have other family members noticed these changes?" asks Dr. J. "She always makes a big deal about things," Ryan mumbles.

The father nods in agreement and adds, "My wife babies the boys." The mother angrily turns on him: "Well if you had grown up in *my* family with *my* brother, you would be hypervigilant too!" Dr. J asks her to explain, and the mother tearfully tells of her brother's slide into alcoholism and chronic mental illness. Dr. J asks the family to comment. Jeffrey and Ryan roll their eyes and look at their father. The father says nothing and the boys look away. Dr. J, noticing this, asks the father directly for his input. The father offers a noncommittal answer.

Dr. J presses the couple. "This is a serious concern. It appears that Mrs. S fears her sons may go down the same path as her brother. What do you all think of this?" Dr. J is careful to use Mrs. S's exact words. With further support, Mr. S eventually states, "My wife exaggerates everything. There is nothing wrong with her brother that good discipline could not have prevented."

Dr. J asks the pertinent question regarding Jeffrey, "Do you disagree about what is wrong with Jeffrey and what needs to happen here?" The father again blames the mother's parenting and states he believes his son needs a firmer hand. The mother again expresses her fears regarding losing her son to alcoholism and tries to talk with Jeffrey about why he is drinking. They had agreed that they disagree and often fight about it. They have never tried to resolve their differences. In this brief exchange about the identifying problem (i.e., Jeffrey's substance abuse), Dr. J has gained valuable information about family history and about the couple's conflict over child rearing. She asks a few more questions about discipline of the children (questions from the behavior control dimension) and the responsibilities and chores of the children at home (from the role allocation dimension).

"Okay, that is important information, but let's focus on Jeffrey. It seems that mother noticed some behaviors first. Who did you tell and what happened then?" Dr. J is exploring problem solving, specifically the communication of the problem to others. The mother responds that she had told her husband, who dismissed it, and then her friend Sally, who encouraged her to tell the pediatrician. A psychological evaluation of Jeffrey has been arranged for Tuesday. The father looks surprised. Dr. J checks in with Ryan, who hadn't noticed anything about Jeffrey and appears to not want to be involved.

Dr. J summarizes the family's problem solving so far. "So, mother noticed some changes, communicated them to father, who dismissed them, and then she took action on her own without discussing it further in the family. Is that correct?" No one responded. Dr. J asked again and all nodded and looked down.

"How do other types of problems get resolved?" Dr. J asks. The family is reluctant to talk. Dr. J gives examples of other areas where problems might arise, such as general repairs around the house or planning vacations. The latter question elicits much discussion from the boys, who get a say in where they go each summer, usually choosing a camping experience, which their mother states she does not enjoy, "but it is three against one." The family then teases her with stories of how they persuaded her to canoe across the lake. The family is now more engaged in the assessment process.

The following is a formal outline of the abbreviated family assessment; while many questions remain to be asked, this brief outline helps with formulating the case and patient management. **(Another example of presenting a formulation to the family is shown on the DVD in scene 13.)**

Problem solving: The couple disagrees on the meaning of Jeffrey's behavior and on parenting in general. The family can identify, communicate, and solve practical problems around the house; however, emotional problems are not identified, communicated, or resolved. The mother overidentifies emotional problems and the father underidentifies emotional problems.

Communication: From what can be observed in the interview, when communication does occur, it is clear and direct. However, there is limited communication between parents and between the children and their parents.

Role allocation: This is a traditional family with the father as the "breadwinner" and the mother as the "homemaker." The boys have no clear chores or responsibilities.

Affective responsiveness: Jeffrey is more aggressive and angry in the past 2 months. Otherwise all family members experience and express a full range of emotion.

Affective involvement: Some information was gained in this dimension when the father and the sons discussed vacations. As far as vacations are concerned, the rest of the family ignores the mother's wishes and interests. The father seems disengaged except around discussion of vacations.

Behavior control: The parents appear to disagree about discipline for the children. This area must be explored next when the family assessment is completed.

Formulation: Summarizing the information and getting corrective feedback is an important part of the assessment process. As this is an abbreviated assessment, Dr. J summarizes the family data in several statements. "So, as I understand things, mother has the major role in child care, identifying and solving problems around the boys, including schooling and health. There is little communication about this as father thinks mother is too lenient but he does not want to take over this responsibility, as he is very busy at work. For other things, like household practical things, both parents communicate freely and agree on what needs to happen. For emotional problems, each member of the family keeps things to themselves, don't communicate emotional problems, and don't discuss emotional problems. Mother, you are generally perceived as overidentifying emotional issues in everyone in the family. Have I got this right?" The family agrees. "In addition, the boys have little responsibility at home, and discipline varies depending on whether mother or father catches them doing something they shouldn't be doing. Is that right?"

As this is an emergency room evaluation, an assessment of Jeffrey's history of presenting symptoms and his mental status must be completed, so Dr. J moves ahead and questions the family about Jeffrey's sleep, eating, school grades, and so on to make a diagnosis and determine level of care. She then asks the family to leave so that she can meet alone with Jeffrey. She starts her interview with Jeffrey by acknowledging that his parents seem to fight about how to manage him and that must be frustrating for him. She thus quickly establishes rapport. He agrees to a short hospitalization "to sort things out" and to try to get his family on the same page about how to work together.

Treatment: In the emergency room, a few specific questions about problem solving provide information about the family dynamics that contribute to Jeffrey's presentation. Understanding Jeffrey in the context of his family gives insight into his likely behavior in treatment. For example, close scrutiny will be interpreted by Jeffrey as a pathologizing gaze "like his mother" and engaging in games and discussions about sports will be interpreted as being "like his father." Thus, even if the family is not amenable, willing, or available to enter treatment, the patient can be understood more easily when the family has been assessed.

It is important to reiterate that a full family assessment must be completed as soon as possible. After a full family assessment, if the family agrees, then family therapy can be part of the outpatient treatment plan. This example illustrates how an assessment can begin in the emergency room and be completed on an inpatient unit, and treatment can begin in the outpatient setting.

Family Assessment in Oncology and Rehabilitation Medicine

Ms. P is a 38-year-old married Hispanic female admitted to the oncology service with a diagnosis of giant cell tumor. She has severe pain and is scheduled for right leg amputation. She is referred to the psychiatrist post surgery because of increasingly withdrawn behavior and refusal to work with the rehab team. She states she is not receiving adequate pain medication.

Psychiatric evaluation identifies a depressive disorder not otherwise specified with significant suicidal ideation. The patient agrees to antidepressant medication. Her husband is present throughout the interview. The interview is completed with an interpreter. Over the next few days, the patient improves and is willing to participate in a family meeting. Her husband, her son, her parents, two sisters and their husbands, and several cousins attend. A young niece, a 24-year-old college junior, wants to act as the family interpreter.

Orientation: Dr. H asks each person to introduce themselves and to state their understanding of the purpose of the meeting. All answers reflected a desire to help the patient. Dr. H indicated that the purpose of the meeting is to discuss Ms. P's psychiatric diagnosis and plans for management of her depression when discharged. Ms. P has not communicated with her family about her depression or her suicidality. Her husband who had been present at the initial interview, is the only member who knows. The patient does not want to bring it up and asks Dr. H to discuss it. The meeting focuses on Ms. P's depressive symptoms and illness management. When asked for a response, the family emphasizes their desire to help and be supportive.

Assessment: The assessment is limited because of time constraints, the large size of the family, and use of an interpreter. Dr. H decides to focus on the extended family's emotional responses to the patient and defers questions about practical aspects of family functioning to a later meeting with the patient and husband. Dr. H asks each family member how he or she feels hearing about Ms. P's thoughts of suicide. Her mother cries, stating she has lost two sons already and asks her daughter "not to think like that." Her father states that he will help her in any way he can. Her 9-year-old son bursts into tears and states that he feels to blame because he had pushed her and she had fallen and hurt her leg and that's why it was cut off. He is inconsolable. No one in the family attempts to comfort him. Eventually his grandfather touches him on the head.

Dr. H spends some time explaining to the family that children often blame themselves for parents' illness and that the boy must be reassured and supported. Dr. H models how to talk with the young boy. An uncle says that he had been suicidal when his back pain was severe and that he understands the patient and reassures her she can feel better. The general response is that the family will watch her and she will not be alone. The patient said she feels that her illness has brought the family together. The husband indicates a major problem is that his wife never tells anyone how she is feeling and is "a private person." All agree and state that she will need to learn to talk more with them. Time did not permit further assessment of the large extended family system. A second appointment is arranged to assess the functioning of the couple and their child.

Problem solving: Questions pertaining to affective/emotional problem solving were asked. Ms. P is unable to communicate affective/emotional problems to her family. Even when an affective/emotional problem presents itself, that is, the son crying inconsolably, the family has limited affective/emotional problem-solving skills.

Communication: Ms. P had difficulty communicating with her family; however, other family members were more open and able to identify and communicate emotional issues.

Role allocation: Assessment deferred to a subsequent meeting.

Affective responsiveness: Dr. H notes that this area needs further evaluation especially regarding the son's tearfulness.

Affective involvement: The family mentions several times that Ms. P will never be left alone. Ms. P expresses her pleasure that her family will be with her at all times. It is unclear if this is a welcome response to the current crisis or if there is any significant concern in this area. Dr. H is aware of needing to assess for cultural aspects to this family's affective involvement.

Behavior control: Assessment deferred to a subsequent meeting.

Formulation: To be done after a full assessment is completed in a subsequent meeting.

Treatment: No specific treatment direction comes from this meeting. Dr. H schedules a follow-up meeting to further assess family functioning, specifically the role differentiation of the couple, taking into account the patient's disabilities. He has so far identified Ms. P's poor affective/emotional communication and the son's tearfulness as two issues of concern. He is also curious about cultural factors in the family's possible overinvolvement with the patient and their lack of response to the young boy's tearfulness.

Family Assessment in the Inpatient Psychiatry Unit

Mrs. S is a 43-year-old white married female with a history of chronic depression, five suicide attempts, and current suicidality. She has been in outpatient treatment by a psychiatrist (who prescribed zolpidem 10 mg at night, quetiapine 100 mg two times/day, escitalopram 20 mg/day, and valproic acid 750 mg two times/day) and a psychologist who was working with her to cope better with the consequences of childhood sexual abuse. Mrs. S has been married for 20 years and has a 19-year-old daughter at home. She has multiple prior hospitalizations and a history of self-injurious behaviors, including cutting, burning, and head banging. She has also been treated with a course of electroconvulsive therapy without significant benefit. She underwent gastric bypass surgery in the previous year, leading to a 150-pound weight loss. Her weight loss led to increased sexual interest by her husband and a reactivation of her anxieties about her sexuality and sexual trauma history. She hates herself and feels hopeless about the future.

During hospitalization, Mrs. S's medications were simplified to escitalopram 30 mg/day as the sole agent. Individual psychotherapy focused on her continued tendency to blame herself for the sexual abuse and the subsequent self-hatred. Initially the patient refused permission for any family meetings, saying that her husband and daughter were fed up with her, her chronic suicidality, and frequent hospitalizations and would therefore not be interested in participating in her current care. She did give consent for the treatment team to contact her husband who, in fact, was more than willing to attend family meetings along with their daughter.

Orientation: During the first meeting Dr. M welcomes the family. "Thank you for coming to this meeting. We try to meet with the families of all of our patients in order to get your ideas about what the problems are, answer any questions that you may have, and plan together what the next steps should be. Is that all right with everyone?" Everyone agrees.

Assessment: The assessment includes a review of everyone's perspectives on the patient's problems and an overview of the family's functioning. Dr. M starts by asking, "How do you understand what the problems are?" The husband and daughter both express frustration with the chronicity of the patient's depression and her hopelessness. They are also very upset, scared, and angry about her repeated attempts to hurt herself. They also, however, express support for and understanding of the issues that she is trying to deal with and an appreciation for her concern and commitment to the family unit.

Problem solving: The family members have good problem-solving skills. They are able to identify, agree upon, and take action to resolve practical problems in their daily lives. They have more difficulties in resolving emotional problems such as the sadness Mrs. S feels and the frustration and anger felt by the husband and daughter.

Communication: They have difficulties communicating, particularly about emotional issues. They are much better at discussing instrumental/ practical concerns.

Role allocation: They allocate roles and responsibilities appropriately. No one feels overburdened, and all necessary family functions are carried out.

Affective responsiveness: The husband and daughter are able to experience an appropriate range of emotions. Mrs. S is consumed with feelings of depression and worthlessness.

Affective involvement: The family is emotionally well connected with each other and caring and supportive most of the time. The patient is surprised at the degree of understanding and support shown by both her husband and daughter. They in turn feel that she truly cares for them and is interested in their welfare.

Behavior control: They have difficulties setting acceptable limits for self-destructive behaviors.

Formulation: Mrs. S has a biological vulnerability to depression. She had been sexually abused as a child, resulting in abnormalities of the hypothalamic-pituitary-adrenal axis. Her depression is not responsive to multiple trials of antidepressants and electroconvulsive therapy. She feels ashamed and guilty about the sexual abuse, feeling that she contributed to its continuation. She feels helpless and hopeless. The recent gastric bypass surgery with its attendant weight loss reactivated conflicts about her sexuality. She has isolated herself from her husband and daughter, convincing herself that they no longer care for her so that she does not have to make continued efforts to cope better with her depression and posttraumatic stress disorder. Her husband's renewed sexual interest in her both pleases and scares her.

Treatment: During the evaluation Mrs. S is pleased to see the degree of concern and support her husband and daughter show toward her. They see her as being very competent in many areas of her functioning. They are able

to engender a sense of hopefulness and connectedness in the patient. The husband and daughter in turn are in agreement with the formulation as outlined
above, feeling that it gives them a better understanding of the various forces
at play in Mrs. S's depression and how they are all trying to deal with it. Issues
concerning the patient's safety and likelihood of future self-harm are discussed. They are able to outline practical steps to take at times when she becomes overwhelmed, such as practicing tolerating the feelings until they pass
rather than feeling a need to act on them, writing down her feelings, letting
the family know how she feels, and contacting her therapist. The husband
and daughter both agree they will continue to be supportive as long as Mrs. S
follows these steps.

A second family meeting is held between the patient and her husband to
discuss the patient's changing body shape and the sexual connotations that
this had for both of them and also how this ties into conflicts that the patient
has been struggling with since her sexual abuse. They are able to discuss and
work out a way of connecting with each other and satisfying the husband's
needs without this being overly threatening to the patient. Mrs. S expresses
appreciation to her husband for his understanding of her concerns and for his
continuing support of her. The husband in turn is able to focus on his wife's
healthy aspects and the value she brings to the family in terms of her intelli-
gence, sense of humor, conscientiousness, and capacity for hard work.

The involvement of the family in this patient's care allows for less reliance
on pharmacotherapy, provides a more focused approach to her resurgent conflict about her sexuality, and facilitates the implementation of a plan that
helps manage her suicidal impulses. She leaves the hospital in better control,
less depressed and more hopeful about the future.

Family Assessment in the Outpatient Clinic

Ms. L is 41 years old, lives alone, and has a history of schizophrenia spanning
two decades. She has had four hospitalizations over the past 20 years and is
on oral neuroleptics. A case manager whom she likes visits her weekly. Her
parents have guardianship. She has a fixed delusion about her father, stating
that she believes he monitors her day and night using video cameras hidden
around her apartment and employs people in the neighborhood to spy on her
when she leaves her apartment. This belief has been investigated several times
over the years by the mental health center and found to be unsubstantiated

and a symptom of her schizophrenia. Ms. L has a close relationship with her mother, who feels torn between her husband and her daughter.

Ms. L presents in an agitated state at the mental health center emergency services with a complaint about her father. She states that he broke into her house and stole money. Her parents are called in as her guardians and to help assess her current mental status and a need for a change in level of care.

Orientation: Dr. M meets with Ms. L and her parents together. "I am Dr. M and I'm going to meet with you today to assess what has been going on and to help decide what needs to happen next. Is that okay?" Mr. and Mrs. L agree. The patient looks suspicious and asks if she is being sent to the hospital. Dr. M repeats that she is going to work with all three of them to decide what should happen next.

Assessment: Dr. M completes an individual assessment and determines that Ms. L has no new psychiatric symptoms and that no change in medication is indicated. She then goes on to assess family functioning.

Problem solving: Father makes all the major decisions about money and gives his daughter grocery money each week, arranges for all maintenance in her apartment and all major purchases. For example, if the refrigerator breaks, Ms. L tells whoever comes by the house first, who then communicates it with her father who then calls the store and arranges for a new refrigerator to be delivered and installed. The father generally provides well, although Ms. L has no input into his decisions. Her parents, chiefly her father, decide whether or not she can accompany them on their annual vacation to Florida. Regarding emotional problems, Ms. L will tell whoever comes by the house first, who then communicates it with her case manager who will visit with her as soon as she can. If it is an issue that involves the parents, the caseworker communicates to the parents, who generally implement her suggestion. Overall, problems get identified and communicated promptly and solutions implemented. Ms. L, however, has no say in this process and is frustrated by this.

Communication: Ms. L communicates clearly when she is in distress, and all three who care for her respond appropriately. There is indirect communication from mother to patient; for example, if the mother does not want to share something with her daughter or take her out, the mother will ask the father to convey that information to her.

Role allocation: Ms. L is expected to keep her house clean although a housekeeper comes once a week. She and her mother go to the grocery store once a week. Ms. L has a fixed amount to spend. Ms. L expresses a desire to be more independent.

Affective responsiveness: Ms. L expresses fear and paranoia and appears to have limited periods of happiness and contentment. Her parents are very anxious and solicitous of her, but this alternates with a heavy-handed prohibition on her desires out of fear that they may be part of her illness.

Affective involvement: The only relationships that Ms. L has are with her parents and the caseworker. Her parents are very involved, helping her decide what she should do and be interested in. Her father comes over to see her unannounced, on his way home from work or late in the evening and usually several times over the weekend. He often calls on the telephone to check on her. He denies driving by her house at night. Her parents express deep concern about what will happen to their daughter when they die.

Behavior control: There are no rules about when the parents can enter her house. They have a key and can decide to stay overnight if they are particularly worried about her.

Formulation: Ms. L's presentation is related to her delusional beliefs about her father. Although Ms. L lives independently, her parents are the major problem solvers, they control many aspects of her life, and their role as guardians underscores the necessity to monitor her at all times. The parents are extremely anxious about their daughter's welfare, now and in the future. Ms. L expresses a desire to be more independent, and the fact that she has delusions about her father controlling her suggests that alternative family arrangements might work better. Ms. L is given the diagnosis of chronic schizophrenia and a parent-child conflict (V61.9 or V61.20 DSM-IV-TR code).

Procedural modifications to a comprehensive assessment of the family

---

- Focus on the most pertinent areas of family functioning
- Obtain the family's agreement about the agenda for the meeting
- Ensure safety for the patient and the family

Treatment: The following immediate plan is agreed to by all involved, including the caseworker. The father will visit only at prescribed times, and the mother will communicate all decisions (good and bad) to the patient. The caseworker will for a short time increase the frequency of home visits, to check on safety and medication compliance. Once a week, Ms. L and the caseworker will meet to discuss future plans (e.g., classes, vacations) and then present these tentative plans to her parents for approval. The patient and caseworker will also work on long-term goals such as developing hobbies, making and budgeting for her own shopping, and cleaning the house. The parents are to think about adding another guardian who would be able to share the responsibility. A meeting is scheduled for later that month with the parents and case manager to review progress.

The caseworker and the parents are involved in a family assessment even though the patient lives alone. Ms. L's elderly parents need help with relinquishing some care, finding another guardian, and being able to enjoy their daughter's company without feeling that they have to control her.

Conclusion

These examples illustrate how an abbreviated assessment of family functioning can be useful in different clinical settings. The examples show that initiating a family assessment that is situation specific can yield important information that can immediately guide treatment. A family assessment can occur at sequential points of care as time and the patient's mental status allow. A complete family assessment must occur before initiation of family therapy.

Reference

1. O'Farrell TJ, Fals-Stewart W: Alcohol abuse. J Marital Fam Ther 29:121–146, 2003

6

Biopsychosocial Formulation

- Neuroscience provides an empirical basis for a biopsychosocial model in psychiatry.
- A good biopsychosocial formulation provides an understanding of the multiple factors related to the presenting problem and ensures that the relevant factors are addressed in treatment.
- A biopsychosocial assessment includes an assessment of family functioning.
- A biopsychosocial formulation shared with the patient and family leads to meaningful dialogue.

What is a biopsychosocial (BPS) formulation, and what does it have to do with families? Family difficulties need to be included in the patient's assessment and treatment in order for treatment to have the best chance of success. The BPS formulation is based on the BPS model as articulated by George Engel (1), who stated that physicians had become insensitive to patients and blamed modern medical training: "The reductionist scientific culture of the day is largely responsible for the public view of science and humanism as antithetical" (p. 538). Engel provided a model that encompasses both the science and the humanism in medicine, integrating the biological, psychological, and sociological aspects of human life. His model is based on general systems theory, which permits scientific investigation across different levels without attempting to reduce higher levels to lower, as the reductionist biomedical model does (2). A systems model states, simply, that one part of the system affects another part of the system and vice versa. Using this systems-theoretical framework, Engel considered difficulties at the psychological, family, or social level, along with the biomedical level, to work out how these factors might interact to produce disease. Engel's model of reciprocal interactive causality replaces the simple cause-and-effect model of linear causality.

Many leaders in psychiatry have challenged the BPS model as being unhelpful in clinical practice and have suggested alternative models. The perspectives model, advocated by McHugh and Slavney (3), discusses psychiatric illnesses from four perspectives: the concept of disease, dimension of character, behaviors, and the concept of the life story. The authors state that a psychiatric illness usually falls into one of these four perspectives, for example, schizophrenia into the disease perspective, personality disorder into the dimensions of character perspective, alcohol abuse into the behaviors perspective, and mild depression or anxiety into the concept of the life story perspective. The perspective model can now be considered a historical model, reflecting the notion that some illnesses were considered biological while other "less severe" illnesses were considered characterological. It also perpetuates the mind/brain split and does not accommodate a view of illness as multifactorial with overlapping etiologies.

More significantly, however, the perspective model does not accommodate recent developments in neuroscience, which show clear neurological correlates of human behavior, normal and abnormal. For example, magnetic resonance imaging identifies brain areas that are active in parenting (4). These areas include the cingulate with feedback loops involving midbrain, basal ganglia, and thalamus for motivation and reward. Other aspects of parenting such as social context and memory processing are activated in other regions including the hippocampus, parahippocampus, and amygdala. Aberrations in these circuits, from whatever cause, affect the parent-child bond, influencing personality development and the future risk for the development of mood and anxiety disorders.

The pluralistic model proposed by Ghaemi (5) emphasizes that no single model can explain the entire field of psychiatry and that the "best model for the job at hand" should be chosen. Thus, a reductionist biological model is appropriate for biological research and a humanistic model is appropriate for dealing with questions about how to live one's life. Most physicians would agree with this, but patients are complex and have illnesses, life situations, and personalities that all affect the presentation of symptoms and the course of their illness. All models might seem entirely reasonable. The pluralistic model does not help the psychiatrist faced with a distraught patient with multiple diagnoses and the patient's worn-out family.

The pragmatic model proposed by Brendel (6) emphasizes evidenced-based treatments. It supports the use of multiple providers, each providing expert treatment in their own area rather than the use of one practitioner who is trained to a basic level in all modalities. The problem with this model is that it assumes the presence of experts in every community and undermines the role of a psychiatrist in providing integrated broad-based treatment. It also presupposes extensive communication and coordination of care between multiple providers, something that is increasingly difficult given the reimbursement and caseload characteristics of the current health care system. As discussed in the introduction, we strongly advocate for the psychiatrist to be adequately trained in multiple modalities, with the ability to refer to a specialist for difficult cases.

Zachar (7) supports the BPS model because it is easy to grasp, intuitive, simple, and a "good enough" working model. It is a folksy model that psychiatrists can keep in their head to refer to when assessing a patient and devising a treatment plan. It also makes sense to patients and their families. If the BPS model acts as a reminder to assess patients fully and to consider all aspects of the patient when developing a treatment plan, then the BPS model has great utility.

Why is the model that psychiatrists work from important? A study that examined the way psychiatrists think about patients showed that the model they used influenced their practice (8). Psychiatrists responded to clinical vignettes and rated the importance of neurobiological, psychological, and social factors in explaining the patients' symptoms. The results showed that the more a behavioral problem was seen as originating in "psychological" processes, the more a patient was viewed as responsible and blameworthy for his or her symptoms. Conversely, the more behaviors were attributed to neurobiological causes, the less likely a patient was viewed as responsible and blameworthy (8). Thus psychiatrists' assumptions about biological or psychological etiological factors influence their assessment and treatment of the patient. For example, unacknowledged assumptions about patients may lead to faulty clinical practice that working with families has no place in the treatment of chronic mental illness or that families cause patients to become ill. The model that physicians use to think about patients has significant effects on their practice. A BPS model clearly encourages a complete assessment and a broad-based treatment plan.

Evidence for the Interaction of Biological, Psychological, and Social Factors

Advances in neuroscience provide the theoretical underpinnings for the BPS model. The following excerpts from major thinkers and researchers explain how biological and psychosocial factors interact. Nobel Prize winner Eric Kandel (9) proposes five principles to be considered in the analysis of the interaction between social and biological determinants of behavior.

Kandel's principles

- **Principle 1:** All mental processes derive from operations of the brain. The actions of the brain underlie all complex cognitive actions, conscious and unconscious.

- **Principle 2:** Genes and their protein products are important determinants of the pattern of interconnections between neurons in the brain and the details of their functioning. Genes, specifically combinations of genes, exert a significant control over behavior.

- **Principle 3:** Altered genes do not, by themselves, explain all of the variance of a given major mental illness. Social or developmental factors are also important contributors. Just as combinations of genes contribute to behavior, including social behavior, so can behavior and social factors exert actions on the brain by feeding back on it to modify the expression of genes and thus the function of nerve cells. Learning, including learning that results in dysfunctional behavior, produces alterations in gene expression. Thus all of "nurture" is ultimately expressed as "nature."

- **Principle 4:** Alterations in gene expression induced by learning give rise to changes in patterns of neuronal connections. These changes not only contribute to the biological basis of individuality but presumably are responsible for initiating and maintaining abnormalities of behavior that are induced by social contingencies.

- **Principle 5:** Insofar as psychotherapy or counseling is effective and produces long-term changes in behavior, it presumably does so through learning, by producing changes in gene expression that alter the strength of synaptic connections and structural changes that alter the anatomical pattern of interconnections between nerve cells of the brain.

The multifactorial origins of psychiatric illness have been teased out by following the trajectory of patients. Michael Rutter (10) summarizes his work with vulnerable children:

> [E]nvironments affect genes—not through effects on genes sequence, but through effects on gene expression. Furthermore, environments affect neuro-endocrine structure, and functioning, and through such effects, may influence brain development. Experiences may affect patterns of interpersonal interaction that become influential through their role in the shaping of later environments; in addition, experiences have to undergo cognitive and affective processing, so that what happens to individuals influences their mental concepts and models of themselves and their environments. (p. 5)

According to Rutter (10), environmental, genetic, and developmental perspectives in an integrated model best describe the pathways to conduct disorder. He integrates these perspectives as follows: Children with certain genetic predispositions are likely to elicit particular reactions from parents and peers. A child who is temperamentally fussy may lead his parents to respond with harsh discipline. The child may bring on his own rejection by peers by behaving in ways that peers find unacceptable. Other factors such as poverty also influence parenting. Over time, parenting, peer experiences, and social experiences alter the child's biological dispositions. Thus, children are born with biological dispositions or into sociocultural contexts that launch them on a trajectory toward conduct problems in later life. These factors tend to direct a child toward particular life experiences, such as harsh discipline, emotional neglect, or conflict with peers and siblings. Eventually, the child acquires relational schemas made up of hostility, aggression, and self-defensive goals. Thus, when confronted with problematic social situations, these children readily make hostile attributions about peers and adults and act aggressively without thinking about consequences. The environment then reacts back to them, usually with hostility and punishment, and a vicious cycle ensues.

Kendler (11) emphasizes the interaction between genetic and environmental risk factors in contributing to major depression. He states:

> Biological reductionists assume that neurobiological risk factors for psychiatric disorders operate through physiological "inside-the-skin" pathways.

However, an emerging body of research suggests that this assumption is false. Part of the way in which genetic risk factors influence the liability to psychiatric disorders is through "outside-the-skin" pathways that alter the probability of exposure to high-risk environments. (p. 437)

Kendler calls his model integrative pluralism because it encourages incorporation of divergent levels of analysis. This approach assumes that, for most psychiatric problems, single-level analyses lead to only partial answers. He adds, "This is not a theoretical issue. If the impact of genetic risk factors is mediated through environmental processes, this opens up new possible modes of prevention" (p. 437).

Does clinical research support the use of the BPS model? Ross et al. (12) illustrated the interaction between biological and psychological factors in the onset of postpartum depression. The variance in depressive symptoms in the perinatal period is best accounted for by the indirect effects of biological risk factors (progesterone) on psychosocial risk factors. The biological risk factor is thought to alter the sensitivity to psychosocial stress and thus determine the threshold for the development of depressive and anxiety symptoms. This study supports a BPS model of disease whereby both biological and psychosocial factors interact to produce disease. Tienari et al. (13) found that in schizophrenia spectrum disorders, adoptees at high genetic risk for schizophrenic spectrum disorders are significantly more sensitive to adverse rearing patterns in their adoptive families compared with adoptees without this genetic risk. In the children with high genetic risk in association with high environmental risk, the incidence of schizophrenia is significantly higher.

How Is a BPS Assessment and Formulation Done?

The development of the BPS formulation is poorly described in the literature. Mechanistic case diagramming to draw linkages between the biological, psychological, and social cultural factors is suggested (14). The aim of this technique is to trace the mechanisms leading from underlying factors such as genetic and social or environmental factors to outward manifestations of illness.

BPS factors assessed

- **Biological:** Biological-genetic vulnerability, comorbid medical/psychiatric illnesses, current medications
- **Psychological:** Meaning of the illness/symptoms, ways of coping and dealing with difficulties, personality style, frustration, impulse control capacity, intellectual functioning, spirituality, insight
- **Social:** Family and interpersonal relationships, social connections and support systems, work functioning, family relationships

---

The integration of traditional psychodynamic factors with biological vulnerability is demonstrated by Summers (15). This formulation addresses the impact of the patient's biological vulnerabilities on the form and content of psychodynamic conflicts. For example, a child with obsessive-compulsive disorder may have intense separation difficulties associated with a strong need for reassurance.

Psychiatry residents are rarely taught how to construct case formulations but report that when they formulated a case using a BPS model, their understanding of their patients increased and they have better supporting information for their diagnoses and treatment plans (16). In this study of 33 psychiatry residents from three different programs, nearly half of the residents report difficulty organizing their data into a formulation or difficulty doing so concisely. Residents indicate that they need to improve in their overall assessment of patients, and they need more experience in formulating cases. The most common problems for those residents who are rated as not competent are a "lack of integration" and a failure to recognize the interplay and impact each component of the BPS model has on the other components.

Residents also have difficulty understanding what BPS psychiatry is. One resident (17) exclaims: "During psychiatry residency, I constantly struggled to learn how to become a biopsychosocial psychiatrist but found little guidance from either the literature or my mentors. Instead, I learned that the excellent practice of psychopharmacology or psychotherapy, by definition, excludes practice of the other. It is well and good to promote research and teaching in combined treatment, but no faculty exists who can teach what has yet to be created" (p. 185). Despite this, the construction of a BPS formulation and treatment plan remains a cornerstone skill for the practicing psychiatrist and a necessary skill to pass the Boards Part II.

How Should Psychiatrists Practice BPS Psychiatry?

Assessment

The BPS approach starts with a thorough assessment. This assessment is a contextualized understanding of the patient within his or her environment and includes an assessment of the patient's significant relationships. BPS components assessed through history gathering are listed in the box at right.

Formulation

A case formulation puts together the above-mentioned aspects of the case and may indicate areas in need of further exploration, for example, lab tests, radiography, psychological/neuropsychological testing, and family meeting. The BPS case formulation is then shared with the patient and family. (**For an example, see scene 13 in the DVD.**) The meaning of the diagnosis and relevant factors, such as medical comorbidity, genetic vulnerability, and cultural issues for this particular patient within the context of the patient's life, are reviewed. It is important to work hard to engage the patient and family, assessing any barriers to engagement and trying to overcome them. Empathic engagement mobilizes the family as allies rather than adversaries in the treatment process. The patient, family, and psychiatrist identify the typical ways the family handles illness and creates meaning around illness. Faulty notions regarding the cause and management of illness can be replaced with explanations that provide for optimal functioning for all family members. Inaccurate patient- and family-driven explanatory models of illness influence clinical outcome. For example, the patient who endorses the notion that hypertension is the consequence of "being tense" will take antihypertensive medicine only when feeling anxious (18). Normalizing emotional reactions to the diagnosis of psychiatric illness can help to allay fears and facilitate a dialogue about the impact of the illness on the patient and family.

Formal BPS presentation

- **Presenting symptoms:** Descriptive, giving DSM-IV-TR differential diagnoses
- **Predisposing factors:** Biological, personality, family functioning, social support
- **Precipitating factors:** Biological, personality, family functioning, social support
- **Mitigating factors:** Biological, personality, family functioning, social support

---

Agreement about treatment should be reached. The psychiatrist lays out treatment options, explaining the rationale and relative merits for each option. The beliefs of the family and their wishes are discussed in depth. This may take several sessions but is the most important part of working with a patient and his or her family. It can prevent future misunderstandings and ensure a good working relationship with both the patient and the family. This expanded assessment, formulation, and sharing of information provides the groundwork for effective treatment. Limitations on time spent with patients and their family for reimbursements from insurance companies have led physicians to compress their interactions with patients and their families into proscribed time limits. This curtails meaningful dialogue about illness and deprives the patient and the family of an important opportunity to understand the illness.

Case Examples

Case 1

Mr. and Mrs. S brought their 17-year-old son, Jeffrey, to the emergency room. Jeffrey was suspended from school after alcohol and marijuana were found in his backpack. The family reports that he has been behaving aggressively at home; he had been withdrawn and, when confronted, becomes angry and belligerent. The parents want him assessed so that he can return to school.

Sharing a BPS formulation

- Establish relationship with patient and family
- Assess and overcome barriers to engagement
- Use empathic engagement to mobilize the family as allies
- Discuss meaning of diagnosis
- Discuss how factors (e.g., medical comorbidity, genetic vulnerability, personality, family, and cultural factors) interact
- Identify family's typical ways of handling illness and their meaning of illness
- Correct inaccurate explanatory models of illness
- Normalize emotional reactions to diagnosis of psychiatric illness
- Lay out treatment options, explaining rationale and merits for each option
- Reach agreement about treatment

Orientation: See Chapter 5, p. 97.

Assessment: This is the complete assessment of the case described in Chapter 5, when the family were first seen in the emergency room.

Problem solving: The couple disagrees on the meaning of Jeffrey's behavior and on parenting in general. The family can identify, communicate, and solve practical problems around the house; however, emotional problems are not identified, communicated, or resolved. The mother overidentifies emotional problems and the father underidentifies emotional problems.

Communication: When communication does occur, it is clear and direct. However, there is limited communication between the parents and between the children and their parents.

Role allocation: The family is a traditional family with the father as the breadwinner and mother as the homemaker. The mother feels burdened with household chores. The boys have no clear chores or responsibilities at home. They are expected to complete their schoolwork.

Affective involvement: The father is disengaged with his wife and his sons except around discussion of vacations. The mother is overinvolved with her sons.

Affective responsiveness: Jeffrey is noted to be more aggressive and angry in the past 2 months. He describes being sad but does not communicate this to others in the family. All other family members experience and express a full range of emotion.

Behavior control: The parents disagree about discipline for the children. The parents agree that Jeffrey should not be using alcohol or marijuana. Otherwise, behavior control is adequate.

Once a complete assessment is done, a full case formulation can be completed.

Case formulation: Jeffrey is an 18-year-old school boy who presents with irritability, sad mood, and withdrawn behavior, meeting criteria for major depressive disorder, mild, and alcohol abuse. There is no past psychiatric history. Predisposing factors include a family history of mood disorder and substance abuse. The major precipitant is conflict with parents about college and the patient's desire to work in his uncle's auto body shop. Jeffrey has an avoidant style and when frustrated leaves the house to visit his uncle. He often does not come home until after midnight and lies to his parents about his whereabouts. Family dysfunction is evident in the vocal parental disputes about child rearing and unsatisfactory division of household chores. Family strengths include a strong sense of family cohesion and parental commitment to child rearing. Treatment options for Jeffrey include the possible use of antidepressants, substance abuse treatment, and further family assessment and treatment to resolve long-standing parental disputes that affect Jeffrey's current functioning. The mitigating factors are that the family is close and overall supportive of each member. Jeffrey's uncle has been communicating with the family and treatment team and is supportive of whatever decision is made.

Formulation to the family: The formulation that was presented to the family at the initial assessment in the emergency room was as follows: "Jeffrey has a type of depression that can respond to antidepressants. He also needs to consider treatment in order to stop drinking. In addition, the way you, as parents, disagree about the rules and expectations has a significant impact on him, and if he is going to get better, you, as parents, will need to come to some agreement about rules and expectations for him. He will also need to learn how to deal more effectively with his frustrations. There may be other family factors that are important too, and these can be explored later. The good things I know about you are that you are a close family, and everyone wants the best for Jeffrey, and Jeffrey, you seem to have a clear idea of what your goals are. What do you think? Do you agree? Anything I have missed?"

Treatment: The family did not immediately respond. The mother asked whether Jeffrey was going to be admitted. The father looked irritated by the question. Dr. J asked Jeffrey if he would consider a short stay to start medication and to give his parents time to meet and work together on family issues. Jeffrey nodded his head, and Dr. J began to describe what would happen next. A few days later, a second family meeting was held to complete the assessment. By that meeting, Jeffrey's parents had drawn up a set of rules for the boys and expected chores and responsibilities. The couple, however, had not addressed their lack of affective involvement. At the end of the family assessment, the couple indicated that they would like help to reestablish closeness in their relationship. Dr. J referred them to a family therapist in the outpatient department. Dr. J continued to work with Jeffrey after his discharge. Dr. J's understanding of the family helped her engage effectively with Jeffrey.

Teaching point: Involving the family in the assessment established the groundwork for future treatment.

Case 2

Ms. L is 41 years old, lives alone, and has a two-decade-long history of schizophrenia. She has had four hospitalizations over the past 20 years and is on oral neuroleptics. A case manager whom she likes visits her weekly. Her parents have guardianship. She has a fixed delusion about her father, stating that she believes he monitors her day and night using video cameras hidden around her apartment and employs people in the neighborhood to spy on her when she leaves her apartment. This belief has been investigated several times over the years by the mental health center and found to be unsubstantiated and a symptom of her schizophrenia. Ms. L has a close relationship with her mother, who feels torn between her husband and her daughter.

Ms. L presents in an agitated state at the mental health center emergency services with another complaint about her father. She states that he broke into her house and stole money. Her parents are called in as her guardians and to help assess her current mental status and a need for a change in level of care.

Orientation: See Chapter 5, p. 106.

Assessment:

Problem solving: The patient's father makes all the major decisions about money and all major purchases. He provides well, although Ms. L has no input into his decisions. Her parents, mostly her father, decide whether or not she can accompany them on their annual vacation to Florida. Ms. L communicates affective issues when she can identify them. If it is an issue that involves the parents, the caseworker communicates to the parents, who generally implement the caseworker's suggestion. Overall, problems, when they are identified, are communicated promptly and solutions are implemented. Ms. L, however, has no say in this process. At times, Ms. L has difficulty identifying emotional problems.

Role allocation: Ms. L is expected to keep her house clean although a home help comes once a week. She and her mother go to the grocery store once a week. Ms. L has a fixed amount to spend. She expresses a desire to be more independent. All family members are pleased and satisfied with the role of the caseworker in monitoring Ms. L's welfare.

Communication: Ms. L communicates clearly when she is in distress, and all three who care for her respond appropriately. There is indirect communication from mother to patient; for example, if the mother does not want to share something with her daughter or take her out, she will ask the father to relay the decision for her.

Affective involvement: The only relationships that Ms. L has are with her parents and the caseworker. Her parents are very involved, helping her decide what she should do and be interested in. Her father comes over to see her unannounced, on his way home from work or late in the evening, and usually several times over the weekend. He often calls on the telephone to check on her. He denies driving by her house at night. Her parents express deep concern about what will happen to their daughter when they die.

Affective responsiveness: Ms. L expresses fear and paranoia and appears to have limited periods of happiness and contentment. Her parents are very anxious and solicitous of her, but this alternates with a heavy-handed prohibition on her desires for fear that they may be part of her illness.

Behavior control: There are no rules about when the parents can enter the patient's house. They have a key and can decide to stay overnight if they are particularly worried about her. Ms. L becomes agitated and more paranoid when the parents stay over, which then increases parental involvement and vigilance.

Case formulation: Ms. L is a 46-year-old single white female with chronic schizophrenia who lives alone and presents with increasing paranoia about her father. Her parents have guardianship. She has had four prior hospitalizations for psychosis and is managed in the community by a case manager who visits her frequently and by a psychiatrist who reports adequate medication compliance. She has a family history of schizophrenia, and her medical history is significant for obesity and non-insulin-dependent diabetes. The major precipitating factor for this presentation is her father's overinvolvement in her life. With all the best intentions to care for his daughter, the father's control of her life and his frequent unannounced visits contribute to her paranoia. Both parents express deep concern about the future welfare of their daughter when they die. The patient expresses resentment toward her parents and wants to have more control over her life. The mitigating factors include a good response to medications and a history of adequate compliance. Ms. L is also motivated for increased self-care and a willingness to work with her family.

Formulation to the family: The formulation is presented to the family as follows: "Ms. L, as you know, you have had a relapse and need to have your medication adjusted. However, one of the major problems is that you feel that you have little control over your life. I understand that you, as parents, have guardianship and need to monitor her closely. However, there will come a time when you are no longer able to care for her and she needs to learn to be as independent as possible. It is really important, Ms. L, to show that you take your medicines regularly. The good things I know about you are that you are a caring family and that Ms. L wants to become independent. What do you think? Do you agree? Anything I have missed?"

Treatment: The parents agreed and suggested that a cousin be invited in to discuss being an alternate guardian. Ms. L wanted to join a local Y and take swimming classes. The caseworker arranged for weekly meetings to continue to help the parents set boundaries around their involvement with their daughter and to facilitate Ms. L as she steps toward more independent living.

Teaching point: Family difficulties negotiating this developmental life stage are important in the presentation of illness. Attention to the family difficulties will substantially reduce the frequency of future relapses.

Biopsychosocial Formulation 123

Case 3

Ms. B is a 22-year-old Cape Verdean female admitted to the hospital with auditory hallucinations telling her to hurt herself. She has had three hospitalizations in the previous 4 months for depression and suicide attempts. The immediate precipitants to this admission are stress from caring for her 16-month-old infant, difficulties in her relationship with her boyfriend, and conflict with her aunt. She does not have a history of substance abuse. She has hypothyroidism that is being treated with thyroid replacement hormones. On admission, she is taking levothyroxine 50 μg, venlafaxine 225 mg, haloperidol 10 mg, quetiapine100 mg, lorazepam 2 mg, and zolpidem 5 mg/night.

Ms. B came to the United States as a child. She reports emotional abuse from her mother leading her to move in with her aunt. She dropped out of school in grade 11 and has been working as a waitress for the past 4 years. She currently lives with her boyfriend, brother, sister, and 16-month-old infant. She has been having problems with her boyfriend, the father of her child, leading to a recent breakup. They have reconciled, against her aunt's advice, but continue to experience difficulties. The reconciliation led to estrangement from her aunt, who was her major source of emotional support and stability.

On admission, the patient shows depressed and anxious mood. Her speech, language, comprehension, and expression are within normal limits. She reports hearing occasional voices but denies visual hallucinations. She thinks that the voices come on when she is under stress and believes they are a reflection of her anxiety and distress. The nature of her stressors and her coping skills are discussed with her. Her antipsychotic and anxiolytic medications are discontinued. She is continued on venlafaxine 225 mg/day. A family meeting is scheduled with the patient, her aunt, boyfriend, and a close girlfriend.

Orientation: It is explained to the family that "the purpose of the meeting is to gain a better understanding of how you all see what the problems are, to give you a chance to ask questions, and to plan together how to proceed after the hospitalization."

Assessment:

Communication: The family has difficulties in discussing issues, especially those that involve feelings. Communication is often indirect, resulting in frustration and misunderstandings.

Problem solving: The family is able to identify problems accurately but is unable to follow through with solutions to deal with them effectively. Even instrumental problems are often unresolved.

Affective responsiveness: The family members report that Ms. B has a pattern of becoming overwhelmed and upset when things do not go her way and that she has a tendency to overreact to small problems. They feel that she is immature and often exhibits attention-seeking behaviors. Ms. B tends to overreact emotionally especially when faced with pressure or the threat of loss of affection.

Affective involvement: All family members feel cared about and connected to others but feel that they do not show this to each other often enough.

Role allocation: Tasks and responsibilities are not well defined or allocated. Ms. B's boyfriend and siblings do not have defined responsibilities in helping to care for their home. They feel that Ms. B is overwhelmed by the responsibility of looking after her daughter and siblings and has difficulty in reaching out for help in a way that allows others to be supportive of her.

Behavior control: There are no clear rules about acceptable behaviors. The boyfriend has cheated on Ms. B and she has attempted to hurt herself on a number of occasions.

Formulation to the family: The formulation is presented to the family as follows: "Ms. B has a biological vulnerability to develop depression and anxiety under stress. She has mixed feelings about needing her aunt and boyfriend to take care of her and her wish to see herself as being able to take care of herself, her daughter, and her siblings without needing others. She does not have good coping skills to deal either with stress or with these mixed feelings. She has unusual experiences when under excessive stress. These experiences also allow her to accept help without admitting to feelings of inadequacy. She takes on too many responsibilities and is not able to accept help from those who could be helpful to her."

Treatment: Family members agree that this formulation is consistent with how they understand the problem. The aunt reiterates her intent to continue to provide emotional support for the patient, as does her boyfriend, but with the condition that she starts to deal with her stresses in a more constructive and proactive manner, including talking to them about her concerns. The boyfriend and her siblings agree to take on specific responsibilities at home. They all decide to talk more openly about their concerns as they come up.

Ms. B agrees to follow up with individual therapy to help with improving coping skills and to deal with her ambivalence. She and her boyfriend express an interest in couples therapy to help them to communicate more effectively. Her mood improves significantly, and she does not have a recurrence of auditory hallucinations.

Teaching point: This case is an example of how a BPS assessment and formulation helped to reframe the patient's problem from being seen as a chronic psychotic condition requiring long-term antipsychotic medications to one that addressed her vulnerability to stress, the pressures in her social situation, her personality style, and her inadequate coping skills to deal with the world. With the new formulation and the help of her family, she was able to see herself not as sick but as overwhelmed. She felt much better about herself and her potential to grow and learn how to deal with her life more effectively while accepting support from those who care for her.

Case 4

Mrs. Y is a 55-year-old mother of three adult children who is admitted to the hospital following an overdose with clonazepam. She has a diagnosis of chronic depression, which has persisted for some 20 years. She is in outpatient treatment with a psychiatrist who has tried many pharmacologic agents with poor results. This is Mrs. Y's fourth hospitalization. Her past inpatient psychiatrist and current outpatient psychiatrist are strongly recommending a course of electroconvulsive therapy. She is currently taking her prescribed medications, which include venlafaxine 150 mg qd, clonazepam 1 mg tid, lamotrigine 100 mg qd, buspirone 10 mg bid, and quetiapine 200 mg qhs.

Mrs. Y meets criteria for major depression. She feels overwhelmed with her responsibilities as a cleaner in a business and with taking care of her husband and a daughter still living at home. A more thorough history of her mood states suggests that she suffers from seasonal affective disorder with euthymia in the summer months. There is a family history of depression in her mother and maternal aunt as well as a nephew who committed suicide. She is healthy except for hypertension, which is well controlled with antihypertensives.

Mrs. Y grew up in Portugal. Her parents were not able to take care of her because they were overburdened by two other sick children and sent her, at the age of 3, to be brought up by an aunt and uncle. She was very upset about being sent away from home initially but quickly came to enjoy the attention and caring in this new family. When she was 11 years old, her parents insisted that she return home to help with the care of her siblings. By this time she wanted to stay where she was and was devastated by having to give up her aunt and uncle's support.

Mrs. Y married a fellow Portuguese worker. They have been married and have lived in the United States for 25 years. They have not learned to speak English very well. Their three adult children speak better English than Portuguese, leading to some estrangement from the parents. Mrs. Y describes a good relationship with her husband and children.

There had been two previous family meetings with other therapists focusing on her medication management, emphasizing the need for compliance with treatments and the advisability of trying a course of electroconvulsive therapy. A family meeting is scheduled to include the patient, her husband, and her three adult children.

Orientation: The family is welcomed to the meeting. It is explained that "family meetings are part of routine care." The family is asked to "outline what problems you are dealing with" and is reassured that "you will have an opportunity to ask questions and that everyone will have the opportunity to be part of deciding what the next course of action should be."

Assessment: The family members describe Mrs. Y as depressed some of the time, focused on herself, and very resistant to change. She derives comfort from her routines (work, as well as cooking and cleaning at home). She does not have outlets outside the home except for visiting a sister who also has depression. The family expresses discontent with her past psychiatric management, which seemed, to them, to consist mainly of trials of different medications. They identify two precipitants to Mrs. Y's current suicide attempt. Her daughter is going through a divorce and Mrs. Y is very worried that her granddaughter may be taken from her mother. This possibility reactivated her unresolved feelings about her separation as a child from her parents and then her aunt and uncle. She is so upset about this topic that she is unable to talk further about how she feels. The other precipitant is the emancipation of her children from home. Without them at home, she feels less needed, less useful, and less meaning in her life.

Communication: Mrs. Y is unable or unwilling to talk about her emotional concerns. Mr. Y is passive and does not talk about emotional issues.

The children are able to communicate about both instrumental and affective issues with each other but not with their parents.

Problem solving: The family is not good at dealing with problems. Mrs. Y avoids dealing with change by reinforcing her routines. Mr. Y is passive and does not get involved in resolving family problems. The children take care of their own issues but do not feel that they can help their parents.

Role allocation: Mrs. Y insists on doing all of the housework in addition to her full-time job. This defines her meaning in life and binds her anxiety. She meets the instrumental but not the affective needs of her family. Mr. Y does as he is asked but does not take any initiatives in the running of the home.

Affective responsiveness: Mrs. Y experiences too much anxiety and sadness. Mr. Y seems underresponsive and disengaged but becomes tearful when discussing family problems, which suggests he has appropriate capacity to experience emotions. The children experience a full range of emotions appropriately.

Affective involvement: The children feel that their mother is selfish and emotionally unavailable to them and their father is caring and supportive but passive. They have become very independent because they felt that they needed to learn to take care of themselves early in their lives.

Behavior control: The family has a clear understanding of acceptable ways of living together. There are no behavioral problems with any family member.

Formulation to the family: The formulation is presented to the family as follows: "Mrs. Y has a biological vulnerability to depression. It runs in the family. This vulnerability has been made worse by early disruptions in her life and undermined her sense of security in being consistently taken care of by adults during her early childhood. She tries to cope with her insecurities, anxiety, and depression by holding to rigid routines, focusing on practical daily tasks, and avoiding dealing with her emotions. Her daughter's divorce and its potential impact on her granddaughter are reactivating unresolved feelings about her own abandonment when she was a young girl. The children's move away from home makes her feel useless and without meaning in her life. Because she has a lot of difficulty in identifying and communicating her feelings so as to provide some relief, this leaves her feeling hopeless and suicidal."

Treatment: The family understands and agrees with the formulation. Mrs. Y agrees that she needs to meet with a therapist to help her to identify and express her feelings more readily and to develop some new interests outside of her home. The family wants the opportunity to meet with a family therapist for follow-up sessions to help them to address their concerns more directly. It is agreed that electroconvulsive therapy is not indicated. Mrs. Y's medication regimen is simplified. The venlafaxine is increased to 225 mg and the other four medications are discontinued as they are not helping. She is started on lithium carbonate 900 mg/day for its potential as an augmenting agent for her current depression and as prophylaxis against seasonal recurrences.

Teaching point: Mrs. Y was seen by her outpatient psychiatrist as having a chronic depression unresponsive to pharmacotherapy and requiring electroconvulsive therapy in addition to polypharmacy. A comprehensive BPS assessment, including meeting with the family, led to a reformulation of the presenting problem. Her treatment now included simplified pharmacotherapy; psychotherapy focused on her sense of vulnerability, difficulty in dealing with emotions, and reestablishing meaning in her life; and family meetings to ensure that nobody felt blamed for the problems and that all had a similar understanding of what steps they could take to minimize the likelihood of these problems persisting. Mrs. Y felt better about being understood and having her feelings validated by those who loved her. She felt more hopeful about being able to take at least some steps that could make her feel better. The family was relieved to have a better understanding of the difficulties they were all dealing with and felt empowered to take some steps of their own to work better together rather than just hoping that some new medical treatment would resolve Mrs. Y's depression.

Conclusion

Biopsychosocial psychiatry now stands on a stronger empirical base as neuroscience illustrates how biological and psychosocial factors interact to produce disease. A BPS formulation enables the psychiatrist to develop a contextualized understanding of the patient in his or her social setting and therefore maximizes the chances of successful treatment. Communication of this formulation to patients and families helps them make sense of the illness and develop a mutual understanding of how the illness can be treated. Engaging the patient and family takes time but lays the groundwork for successful family-oriented care.

McLaren (19) states that "unless there is an integrating theory already in place, gathering biological, psychological and sociological data about people will only yield scattered lumps of information that do not relate to each other in any coherent sense. Without an overarching theory to integrate the fields from which the data derive, associations between different classes of information are meaningless" (p. 91). A biopsychosocial approach to integrating the elements in a formulation provides the psychiatrist, the patient, and the family with a mutual understanding of the patient in their context. This understanding provides the basis for a BPS treatment plan.

References

1. Engel GI: The clinical application of the biopsychosocial model. Am J Psychiatry 137:535–544, 1980
2. Bertalanffy LV: General Systems Theory: Foundations, Development, Applications. New York, Braziller, 1968
3. McHugh PR, Slavney PR: The Perspectives of Psychiatry, 2nd Edition. Baltimore, MD, Johns Hopkins University Press, 1998
4. Swain JE, Lorberbaum JP, Kose S, et al: Brain basis of early parent-infant interactions: psychology, physiology, and in vivo functional neuroimaging studies. J Child Psychol Psychiatry 48:262–287, 2007
5. Ghaemi SN: Paradigms of psychiatry: eclecticism and its discontents. Curr Opin Psychiatry 19:619–624, 2006
6. Brendel D: Healing psychiatry: a pragmatic approach to bridging the science/humanism divide. Harv Rev Psychiatry 12:150–157, 2004
7. Zachar P: The biopsychosocial model: strengths versus weaknesses related to assumptions about good scientific categories. Paper presented at the 158th annual meeting of the American Psychiatric Association, Atlanta, GA, May 2005
8. Miresco MJ, Kirmayer LJ: The persistence of mind-brain dualism in psychiatric reasoning about clinical scenarios. Am J Psychiatry 163:913–918, 2006
9. Kandel ER: A new intellectual framework for psychiatry. Am J Psychiatry 155:457–469, 1998
10. Rutter M: How the environment affects mental health. Br J Psychiatry 186:4–6, 2005

11. Kendler KS: Toward a philosophical structure of psychiatry. Am J Psychiatry 162:433–440, 2005

12. Ross LE, Sellers EM, Gilbert-Evans SE, et al: Mood changes during pregnancy and the post-partum period: development of a biopsychosocial model. Acta Psychiatr Scand 109:457–466, 2004

13. Tienari P, Wynne C, Sorri A, et al: Long-term follow-up study of Finnish adoptees. Br J Psychiatry 184:216–222, 2004

14. Guerrero AP, Hishinuma ES, Serrano AC, et al: Use of the mechanistic case diagramming technique to teach the biopsychosocial-cultural formulation to psychiatric clerks. Acad Psychiatry 27:88–92, 2003

15. Summers RF: The psychodynamic formulation updated. Am J Psychother 57:39–51, 2003

16. McClain T, O'Sullivan PS, Clardy JA: Biopsychosocial formulation: recognizing educational shortcomings. Acad Psychiatry 28:88–94, 2004

17. Lissak M: Biopsychosocial psychiatry. Am J Psychiatry 160:185–186, 2003

18. Kleinman A: Patients and Healers in the Context of Culture. Berkeley, University of California Press, 1988

19. McLaren N: A critical review of the biopsychosocial model. Aust NZ J Psychiatry 32:86–92, 1998

7

Diagnostic Reasoning and Clinical Decision-Making Process

- Explain the rationale for involving families in the decision-making process.
- Explore the meaning of the diagnosis for the patient and family.
- Engage the patient and family in decision making. Normalizing family reactions to the diagnosis and management of psychiatric illness can help establish a good working relationship with the patient and the family. Psychiatrists need to understand why some families are hostile and then work to reduce and manage any hostility. Psychiatrists must appreciate the caregiving role and offer additional support for caregivers if needed.
- Discuss treatment options. It is important to socialize the patient and family to the variety of treatment paradigms such as the provision of medications and psychotherapy (individual and/or family). Patients and families appreciate understanding how different approaches (such as cognitive-behavioral therapy or psychopharmacology) view illness and symptoms differently.
- After a plan is agreed on, the psychiatrist should meet with the patient and family to follow up on how the plan is being implemented, to check on problems, and to make sure everyone still agrees with the plan.

Diagnostic reasoning and clinical decision making are perhaps the most intellectually stimulating aspects of providing clinical care. After gathering information, the physician has to decide how to put the information together to develop a comprehensive formulation and how to construct the most elegant

131

and effective treatment plan. As more proven and effective treatments become available, the opportunities to help become more exciting. Generally speaking, diagnostic reasoning and clinical decision-making occur as a process. This process depends on the site of evaluation. In the emergency room, the purpose of the interview is to establish a provisional diagnosis and decide on a level of care. An inpatient formulation is much more extensive and is the basis for a comprehensive treatment plan that will be mostly carried out in the outpatient setting. The interview of a consultation liaison psychiatrist differs from that of a psychodynamic psychiatrist in private practice. Most initial interviews focus on making a multiaxial diagnosis, but beyond that, psychiatrists' approaches to patients can differ markedly. Psychiatry is unlike most other branches of medicine in that one's training and philosophy of care can be determinants of the treatment the patient receives.

Training informs the psychiatrist's diagnostic reasoning and decision-making skills. A psychiatrist who has been trained biologically will perform a diagnostic interview, prescribe a medication, and use a research evidence–based medication algorithm. A psychiatrist with training in systems theory will assess a patient in his or her family system and assess family functioning in addition to establishing a DSM diagnosis. An individual psychotherapist reviews early childhood experiences and develops a psychodynamic explanation for the patient's symptoms. Learning biological psychiatry is easier than learning psychodynamically based psychiatry, which requires the trainee psychiatrist to experience initial feelings of uncertainty and lack of mastery (1). Learning to be competent and comfortable in performing family assessments and interventions may be equally difficult. Good teachers and role models are essential to mastering these important humanistic aspects of psychiatric assessment and care. This chapter outlines the clinical process of decision making in family-oriented patient care.

Putting the Biological Paradigm in Its Place

The prevailing paradigm in psychiatry is biological: the patient has a DSM diagnosis for which there is a medication and a pharmacologic algorithm if monotherapy fails. This may be partly due to health insurance companies' limiting reimbursement and partly to results from medication trials funded by the pharmaceutical industry. There are several major critiques citing the inadequacy of these medication trials in their application to the broader psychiatric population. First, the patients enrolled in randomized controlled trials in psychiatry usually have one disorder (e.g., major depression), unlike patients in real practice who commonly have several disorders (e.g., depression, anxiety, substance abuse). Second, follow-up in research studies of pharmaceutical agents is often short term (weeks), whereas the actual treatment of psychiatric illnesses are usually long term (years) as these disorders are in most cases chronic or relapsing. Third, treatment outcome studies, for instance for depression, are often efficacy trials rather than effectiveness trials. As such, they examine a homogeneous and unrepresentative sample of patients with depression. Outcome data from such studies most likely overestimate response rates (2). For example, Keitner et al. (3) reported that only 27 (7%) of 378 responders to advertisements for depression treatment studies met eligibility criteria for participation in those studies. Similarly, Zimmerman et al. (4) found that only 29 (8%) of 346 outpatients with depression would have qualified for participation in an antidepressant efficacy trial given the common exclusion criteria that are used in clinical trials. Patients and families need to be educated about the limitations of some research findings.

The mismatch between clinical trials and the realities of actual patients occurs because the majority of clinical trials are mainly designed for a business purpose—to achieve regulatory approval, and thus market access. For many patients, the interactions between multiple medical conditions and multiple interventions over time are complex and difficult to capture in research studies. Finally, the meaning and personal experience of living with a psychiatric illness are not captured in a clinical trial. Most patients and families are unaware of the mismatch between clinical drug trials and the reality of illness experience.

Limitations of the biological paradigm

- Has too narrow a focus
- Downplays the importance of psychological and social influences
- Leads to overreliance on pharmacotherapy

Rationale for Involving Families in the Decision-Making Process

Family research gives a clear scientific rationale for involving families in patient care. Family factors influence the course of psychiatric illness. Patients with major depression who have significant family dysfunction have a slower rate of recovery (5, 6). Conversely, good family functioning is identified as one of five factors that improves outcome in major depression (7). High levels of criticism, hostility, or emotional overinvolvement are associated with relapse in many psychiatric illnesses (8), such as schizophrenia, depressive disorders, acute mania, and alcoholism. How a family member perceives mental illness can also play an important role in the patient's relapse. Relatives who are more critical are more likely to hold patients responsible for their actions rather than attribute their behavior to the illness (9).

Families want to be involved in patient care and want care that focuses on building rapport and communication (10). Families identify several problems with current approaches to treatment, such as conflict with health professionals about treatment and lack of a role for families in the treatment of their relatives. African American families identify isolation of their communities from the mental health care system. Adolescents emphasize that they also are caregivers and identify their need for support. Family members state that they benefit from help that focuses on specific problems, such as how to manage disruptive patient behavior. The National Alliance on Mental Illness recommends improved collaboration between provider, consumer, and family (11). Families want psychiatrists to work with them to establish partnerships that promote an atmosphere of mutual respect; respect the needs, desires, and concerns of families; include families in decisions that involve them; and develop mutual goals for treatment and rehabilitation (12). Families also want psychiatrists to teach them skills to cope with the illness.

Treatment can proceed more smoothly when the patient, the family, and the treatment team have the same understanding of the diagnosis and illness. The implementation of this aspect of care is one of the most understudied in psychiatry. Psychiatrists are aware of the work of cultural psychiatrists, of psychologists who are experts in attribution theory and communication, and of the work on poor medication compliance, yet psychiatry has not found a way to integrate this knowledge adequately into daily practice. The psychiatrist, patient, and family, after discussion about attitudes to illness and care, can reach an agreement about acceptable treatments. This lays the foundation for successful treatment with less likelihood of resistance to care.

Meaning of a Diagnosis

A diagnosis allows patients and families access to services and care. A diagnosis allays fears by giving a name to experiences, such as suicidal thoughts or hallucinations that are frightening to patients and their families. However, a psychiatric diagnosis can be stigmatizing. Counteracting the stigma are current expectations that pharmacological treatments will cure these illnesses. Television advertising and pharmaceutical industry literature, while providing hope for patients, also offer false promises. As many patients and families will attest, a biomedical approach to psychiatric illnesses has limitations.

A DSM diagnosis can be misleading because a patient's experience of psychiatric illness is not as discrete as DSM describes. The DSM diagnostic system is based on consensus and not experimental evidence. Designated experts divide psychiatric disorders into discrete categories based on discussion and consultations. DSM does provide a vocabulary for practicing psychiatrists but perpetuates a categorical, discontinuous view of psychiatric illness. In reality, comorbidities are high and there is a propensity for one condition to merge into another. DSM categories are also frequently undergoing revision, for example, the introduction of spectrum diagnoses in bipolar disorder and schizophrenia in DSM-IV-TR (13). In addition, detection of prodromal symptoms of illnesses, which are not included in DSM-IV-TR diagnoses, are very important in preventing illness relapse.

No objective tests exist to help clarify and consolidate psychiatric diagnoses. Thus diagnoses in psychiatry are less firm than in other areas of medicine. Diagnostic and therapeutic procedures are less focused on critical momentary decisions and more focused on a gradual, iterative procedure. Psychiatric treatments, especially psychotherapy, are self-referencing processes, in which assessments and decisions are constantly reevaluated. These concepts need to be made explicit to patients and families to prevent misunderstandings.

Reaching a diagnosis can be presented as a process that occurs over time, and meanings associated with the diagnosis are evaluated as new information emerges about the illness. The challenge for health professionals and support organizations is to acknowledge medical uncertainty in an atmosphere that allows lay knowledge and expertise to be recognized and discussed. Uncertainties can be resolved in a supportive and open forum in order for the patient and the family to make sense of the diagnosis and move forward with effective adapting and coping strategies. Diagnosis is a rubric for patients, families, and doctors to use as a road map to plan treatment.

Causal Attributions by Patients

How do patients conceptualize illness and symptoms? Symptom experience is embedded in personal, familial, and cultural systems of meaning, and many competing schemas can be present (14). A patient who has a depressive disorder can believe that the illness is "punishment for past wrongdoing" and simultaneously understand that the illness is caused by a "chemical imbalance." The relative prominence of competing explanations is determined by the social context. In the hospital, the patient may agree with the prevailing "chemical imbalance" explanation, perhaps to please the treatment team. When the patient goes home, the prevailing family belief may be that the depression is "punishment for past wrongdoing," and the patient is less likely to continue with the medications.

Family experiences thus serve as examples of illness experience. For example, when a patient's father who became psychiatrically ill recovered without medication, the patient subsequently refused to take medication and believed that, like his father, he could get better without medication. This led to multiple hospitalizations and a serious suicide attempt, which the patient interpreted as being unable to live up to his father's example of self-reliance in recovery. Understanding the explanations that are embedded in the family history, if made explicit, can result in successful treatment.

Patients may enter a clinical setting with clear ideas about the nature of their illness. They may say they have bipolar disorder based on their reading or research on the Internet. Patients may request certain medications based on drug company literature and their side effect profile rather than their relative efficacy. A patient may say, "My brain has a chemical imbalance, and I need drug X to correct the imbalance." Another patient may say that he knows that there is a chemical imbalance in his brain, but he fears that drugs will change his personality and he refuses medication. Another patient may say, "I worry constantly and can't seem to relate to others" and be ambivalent about trying either medication or psychotherapy. Some patients come to treatment requesting only "natural" herbal remedies. Some patients demand electroconvulsive therapy whereas some are terrified of the thought of it. Patients may also have faulty notions regarding the management of illness (15). Another patient may say "My family is driving me crazy" and demand a family meeting. Others may refuse family meetings out of frustration, anger, or fear of disappointment in not having family members as available for support as they hope.

Why Involve families in treatment planning?

- Families want to be involved
- Family functioning influences the outcome of psychiatric disorders
- Therapists and families see opportunity to correct misconceptions
- Therapists and families can create better collaboration, support, and compliance

Case Example

Mr. B is admitted to an inpatient psychiatric unit with severe depressive symptoms including agitation and difficulty sleeping. He focuses almost exclusively on his family not being supportive of him as the root cause of his symptoms. A family meeting is called for the day after his admission. Mr. B is delighted to have his whole family present. He states that he believes all family members should love each other and get on well. If his family did that, he states, then he would feel well. It is soon clear that Mr. B holds unrealistic expectations of what family life should be like. He had grown up in an orphanage and idealizes family life. He cannot understand it when his daughter and his second wife state that they choose to "agree to disagree about many issues." The family meeting clarifies to him that all his family (wife, adult daughter, and four adult sons) and the treatment team acknowledge that his expectations are unrealistic and that he cannot change how others think and behave. It is also clear that he needs to be treated with an antidepressant but he had refused for many years, believing that the family conflict was the cause of his problem. His family, with the support of the psychiatrist, encourage him to take medication. Successful treatment could only begin when the meaning of his illness was addressed. His treatment begins with an exploration of his belief system and a family meeting, and then biological treatment is initiated. The process is a true integrated approach that utilizes elements of many different modalities. In fact, it is often hard to identify where assessment and treatment begin and end in this initial phase of understanding the patient, his family, and his presenting problems. In all cases, the clinician must begin with an understanding of the patient's and family's views about illness and treatment and include education about the illness as part of the treatment.

Causal Attributions of Family Members

Possession by evil spirits and environmental pollution are the most commonly reported esoteric causes of psychiatric illness. More than 50% of family members reported at least one esoteric factor among the possible causes of chronic psychiatric illness (16). Each of the six esoteric causes (possession by evil spirits, environmental pollution, lack of vitamins, punishment by God, radiation, and unfavorable horoscope) was endorsed as likely or very likely by some family members. In addition, nearly 20% believed that there were multiple esoteric causes of their relative's illness. Many of the family members endorsed family-related factors as causes of schizophrenia; 63.9% of participants reported one or more family-related factors as a cause and 44.3% reported two or more family-related causes. These factors include hostile or rejecting attitude of parents, broken home, father too severe, lack of parents' love, too high expectations of parents, and overprotective mother. These unexpectedly high percentages may be a vestige of earlier family-blaming theories of schizophrenia.

Attributional variables are reliable predictors of relapse of schizophrenia at 9-month follow-up (9). When family members attribute problem behaviors in their relatives as internal to and controllable by them, this leads to attempts to coerce the relative "to get back to normal." A critical attitude then develops with family members becoming angry at the relative's willfulness and refusal to try harder. Family members who understand that their relative's behavior is symptomatic of a biological illness called schizophrenia are much less critical of the patient. Looking at attributions (i.e., how the family members understand the patient's symptoms) is therefore an important part of the assessment process.

Engaging Patient and Family in Decision Making

Engagement is facilitated when each family member is individually addressed and listened to. Families may express a sense of failure as they acknowledge their inability to resolve family problems and may express guilt or blame themselves for their relative's illness. In a family meeting, family members may be anxious as they anticipate being discussed, criticized, and confronted. Families express several needs: to be included in the care of their relative, to be understood, and to be respected as concerned relatives who are doing the best they can.

(Scene 3 of the enclosed DVD illustrates clearly how to explore the presenting problem and how to engage each family member.)

Physicians may avoid meeting with the family if they do not have a definitive diagnosis and treatment plan because they do not want to be seen as unsure or unprepared, but the willingness to reach out to a family is reassuring and seen as supportive and caring. Being straightforward with the family about the need to gather information is acceptable to most family members. It is preferable to meet with the family for a short time to explain the diagnostic process because this will help engage the family and establish a collaborative relationship.

Normalizing emotional reactions and family or life stage transitions often allays unfounded fears. For example, after the birth of a child, the family needs to reorganize to include a third person. A mother with postpartum depression may need her husband to become the primary caregiver with their infant during her recovery process. Her husband may have difficulty understanding what that role means if he has not had a good parental role model. The process of discussing normal life stage transitions helps to untangle the issues and can occur over several sessions.

Engaging the hostile family

- Do not avoid them
- Recognize that a hostile family is not necessarily dysfunctional
- Validate the stress and helplessness that the family may be experiencing
- Focus on strengths in the family
- Be sensitive to different cultural norms and expectations

Engaging the Hostile Family

It is hard to engage angry and hostile family members. Some family members may have had negative experiences with the mental health system and feel angry about being blamed or incriminated in the patient's illness. Other family members may be angry because they do not believe in mental illness and see the patient as just lazy (17). A common mistake made by psychiatrists is the avoidance of the hostile family (18). Most families have been on the frontlines providing care, support, and advocacy for their mentally ill family member. The angry family may have been ignored or mistreated by the mental health system in the past. The hostile family is not necessarily dysfunctional. Family members are often angry and upset because of feelings of helplessness. It is helpful for the psychiatrist to recognize how stressful it is for families to deal with a psychiatrically ill relative and to be compassionate toward the difficult family member. Being mindful and looking for strengths is helpful for the family, the patient, and the treatment team. For example, attending a meeting may be difficult for some families because of transportation problems and work schedules, thus their coming together for a meeting can be acknowledged as a family strength. Acknowledging this strength can be the foundation of a good working alliance.

Culture and Ethnicity

Every family has its own individual set of rules and beliefs, which can influence the family's willingness to work with the treatment team. Obvious differences occur across different sociocultural groups, and an open acknowledgment of these differences between the treating physician and the family promotes a working alliance. There are many varieties of family beliefs, and it is important that these beliefs or cultural norms do not get mislabeled as pathological. Ways of interacting and expressing conflict vary widely among families and across cultures. How emotion is expressed, for example, can vary widely and can influence a family's discussion of conflictual issues. A display of great emotion may be needed in some families to illustrate the seriousness of a situation. Deference to older family members in Asian cultures and emotional constriction in some northern European cultures can interfere with conflicts being openly acknowledged and discussed. When psychiatrists meet with a family, asking them what the norms within the family are allows the family to educate the psychiatrists about that particular family's ways of doing things (19).

Differences in culture and/or ethnicity between physician and patient can contribute to poor communication. For example, Korean American and Mexican American patients are reported to have less need for information and participation in decision making than white American patients. Furthermore, patients from different European countries attach different importance to various communication aspects, such as the amount of biomedical and psychosocial communication they consider important. For Chilean patients, being touched by their doctor is an important attribute, but British patients do not mention this as a valuable quality (20).

People belonging to sociocentric cultures see themselves as part of the family, with less emphasis on individuality. Asians are therefore less likely to be assertive and direct in their conversations than Americans, who are focused more on themselves as individuals. In sociocentric societies, emotional over-involvement is to be expected because the individual is seen as part of a close-knit family group. In Indian and in Jewish families, it is culturally acceptable and not considered pathological for mothers to be very involved with their sons. When families migrate, the influence of the "new culture" has different effects on each family member, usually with the younger members becoming more acculturated. There may be internal conflicts in the family based on split loyalties related to the "traditional" or "old" ways versus the "new" ways. The psychiatrist can easily elicit these differences by direct enquiry.

Understanding Caregivers

Family caregivers of relatives with chronic psychiatric illness report depressive symptoms and impaired social, family, physical, and emotional functioning (21). These difficulties are collectively referred to as *caregiver burden*, the way in which a caregiver's lifestyle has been altered by her or his role as a caregiver. *Objective burden* describes the effects of caregiving on the health, finances, and activities of the caregiver; *subjective burden* is the extent to which relatives feel burdened and includes worrying, tension, insomnia, and resentment.

Caregivers who understand that their relative's behavior is caused by illness and not by willfulness report the least burden (22). Psychoeducational interventions for caregivers that improve the caregiver's knowledge of the illness reduce caregiver subjective burden (23, 24). Caregiver quality of life also improves with services that support, educate, and involve family members (25). When caregivers receive emotional support from family and friends, especially the knowledge that other families struggle with similar problems, they develop a stronger sense of family competence (26). The psychiatrist can be helpful in understanding the caregivers' struggles and can be instrumental in helping the caregiver access needed support and services.

Discussing Treatment Options

Patients and families are often unsure what treatments are available and what treatments work. In addition, there are a variety of treatment paradigms such as the provision of medications alone, the provision of psychotherapy alone (individual/family), or the combination of both that the patient/family/psychiatrist might prefer. A family psychiatrist advocates for the inclusion of the family in the process of decision making and treatment planning, discussing the risks and benefits of each treatment option with the patient and the family. This discussion should include the studies that show the impact of providing these treatments alone or in combination. It is important to discuss all treatment approaches that have been shown to be effective for that illness. Family members often find information on the Internet advocating one treatment approach over another. The psychiatrist needs to examine the source and the evidence presented and take the family members seriously, recognizing their efforts as aimed at helping their relative who is ill, not questioning the psychiatrist's judgment. Patients and families appreciate understanding how different approaches (such as cognitive-behavioral therapy or psychopharmacology) view illness and symptoms differently.

Discussing treatment options with the family

- Review the risks and benefits of each treatment with the family
- Recognize that many family members may be well informed through Internet searches
- Try to identify the leading element (rate-limiting process) in the family

---

The Concept of the Leading Element

Systems theory includes the notion of a leading element, which is analogous to the rate-limiting step in an experiment. It is the critical "make or break" aspect of a case—the element of a case that needs to be addressed first. For example, it is common wisdom that alcohol abuse/dependence needs to be addressed before any other aspect of a case; thus, alcohol abuse is considered the starting point of treatment and the leading element. Other examples might include the belief that the illness is caused by evil spirits, and a religious or spiritual consultant may need to be invited to work with the family before psychiatric treatment can begin. If the patient is convinced that her spouse wants a divorce, then that aspect of the case needs to be assessed before recovery can begin. The leading element is best identified during the assessment but may only be uncovered when the case does not go well, or when there is resistance to treatment. After a plan is agreed upon, meeting with the patient and family to follow up on how the plan is being implemented, to check on problems, and to make sure everyone still agrees with the plan is an important part of follow-through.

Case Example

Ms. C has bipolar disorder and has been stable on lithium carbonate for 8 years. Recently she has become aware that her husband has been making business decisions without including her and realizes that she has no knowledge of their current financial status. She is anxious about their financial planning, but attempts to discuss this with her husband have been unsuccessful. She became very angry when she found out that a business deal that she had no knowledge of had fallen through. She brought her husband to the next therapy session and stated that if he didn't start including her in the financial decisions, she didn't think the relationship was viable. Dr. J listened and suggested that they both come back for a couples assessment and booked them for an hour the following week. At that visit, the following information was gathered.

Problem solving: Ms. C handled all of the instrumental problem solving around the house. Mr. C took care of financial issues. They tended to operate as individuals and not communicate much about these areas. They were successful in managing their individual domains. They spent no time discussing future plans.

Communication: Little communication occurred. During the session, the couple found it hard to talk with each other, often using indirect and masked communication.

Role allocation: Ms. C took care of the house and child care. Mr. C brought home the money and employed a gardener to take care of the landscaping. They each took their own car into the garage for repairs. Ms. C attended to the children and their schooling. Mr. C was peripherally involved with the children.

Affective involvement: They did little together, as Mr. C was busy with his work and Ms. C was busy caring for the children.

Affective responsiveness: Mr. C said that he was a very emotional person but didn't express any feelings. He said he was afraid of involving his wife in any business decisions as she had become manic when he had involved her the last time. He said his wife seemed always angry with him, and he was afraid sometimes to come home and tended to avoid her. Ms. C agreed that she was often angry and blamed her husband for causing her to be angry. She agreed that her husband was not able to express feelings and that he was "constricted."

Behavior control: No problems were identified in this area.

The couple agreed with this assessment and was eager to try to work on their problems. Dr. J discussed how that would happen. Both Mr. and Ms. C felt that Dr. J would be able to be fair despite being Ms. C's physician for 3 years. After two sessions of couples work, it was clear that the therapy had stalled. In the discussion about this, Mr. C stated that he found he had a real problem with expressing his feelings. The couple and physician discussed options and decided that individual therapy might help Mr. C. He went to an individual therapist for approximately six sessions, and then the couple came back for couples therapy. After three further sessions, the couple had improved functioning and agreed that the goals of treatment had been reached. The couples therapy ended, and Ms. C continued with medication visits. This case illustrates the need for continuous assessment and decision making and flexibility in choosing treatment.

Best Practice for Clinical Decision Making

Physicians, especially psychiatrists, need time to comprehensively assess their patients. They need time to think about and contemplate the range of factors that contribute to the patient's problems and time to apply good clinical reasoning in formulating the case. Psychiatrists must understand psychodynamic theory as well as neuroscience to understand relevant psychodynamic issues as they relate to the patient's problems. According to Philip Boyce (27), trainees need "the opportunity to work with, observe and discuss good practice. They need to have time to discuss cases with senior clinicians so that they can make use of, and incorporate their experience and so develop the wisdom required of a good psychiatrist" (p. 6). As reimbursement for treatment has become less generous, more patients have to be seen in a shorter time. There is less time to think and reflect on patient problems and less time to teach.

Best practice means performing a comprehensive assessment, making sure the patient and family understand the illness adequately to ensure that they can make an informed decision about treatment. Best practice means that patients and families understand the illness, the course of illness, the impact of different treatment options, and the implications of care delivered by one or multiple practitioners.

References

1. Luhrmann T: Of Two Minds: The Growing Disorder in American Psychiatry. New York, Knopf, 2000
2. Parker G, Anderson IM, Haddad PC: Clinical trials of antidepressant medications are producing meaningless results. Br J Psychiatry 183:102–104, 2003

3. Keitner GI, Posternak MA, Ryan CE, et al: How many subjects with major depressive disorder meet eligibility requirements of an antidepressant efficacy trial? J Clin Psychiatry 64:1091–1093, 2003

4. Zimmerman M, Mattia JI, Posternak MA: Are subjects in pharmacological treatment trials of depression representative of patients in routine clinical practice? Am J Psychiatry 159:469–473, 2002

5. Keitner GI, Miller IW: Family functioning and major depression: an overview. Am J Psychiatry 147:1128–1137, 1990

6. Miller IW, Keitner GI, Whisman MA, et al: Depressed patients with dysfunctional families: description and course of illness. J Abnorm Psychol 101:637–646, 1992

7. Keitner GI, Ryan CE, Miller IW, et al: Recovery and major depression factors associated with twelve-month outcome. Am J Psychiatry 149:93–99, 1992

8. Butzlaff RI, Hooley JM: Expressed emotion and psychiatric relapse. Arch Gen Psychiatry 55:547–552, 1998

9. Barrowclough C, Hooley JM: Attributions and expressed emotion: a review. Clin Psychol Rev 23:849–880, 2003

10. Rose LE, Mallinson RK, Walton-Moss B: Barriers to family care in psychiatric settings. J Nurs Scholarship 36:39–47, 2004

11. Marshall TB, Solomon P: Releasing information to families of persons with severe mental illness: a survey of NAMI members. Psychiatr Serv 51:1006–1011, 2000

12. Lefley HP: Family Caregiving in Mental Illness. Thousand Oaks, CA, Sage, 1996

13. American Psychiatric Association: Diagnostic and Statistical Manual of Mental Disorders, 4th Edition, Text Revision. Washington, DC, American Psychiatric Association, 2000

14. Young A: Rational men and the explanatory model approach. Cult Med Psychiatry 6:57–71, 1982

15. Kleinman A: Patients and Healers in the Context of Culture. Berkeley, University of California Press, 1988

16. Esterberg ML, Compton MT: Causes of schizophrenia reported by family members of urban African American hospitalized patients with schizophrenia. Compr Psychiatry 47:221–226, 2006

17. Brewin CR, MacCarthy B, Duda K, et al: Attribution and expressed emotion in the relatives of patients with schizophrenia. J Abnorm Psychol 100:546–554, 1991

18. Heru AM, Drury L: Working with families of psychiatric inpatients. Baltimore, MD, Johns Hopkins University Press, 2007

19. Dyche L, Zayas LH: The value of curiosity and naiveté for the cross-cultural psychotherapist. Fam Process 34:389–399, 1995

20. Schouten BC, Meeuwesen L: Cultural differences in medical communication: a review of the literature. Patient Educ Couns 64:21–34, 2006

21. Heru AM, Ryan CE: Burden, reward, and family functioning of caregivers for relatives with mood disorders: 1-year follow-up. J Affect Dis 83:221–225, 2004

22. Wendel JS, Miklowitz DJ, Richards JA, et al: Expressed emotion and attributions in the relatives of bipolar patients: an analysis of problem solving interactions. J Abnorm Psychol 109:792–796, 2000

23. Dixon L, Stewart B, Burland J, et al: Pilot study of the effectiveness of the family-to-family education program. Psychiatr Serv 52:965–967, 2001

24. Reinares M, Vieta E, Colom F, et al: Impact of a psychoeducational family intervention on caregivers of stabilized bipolar patients. Psychother Psychosom 73:312–319, 2004

25. Corring D: Quality of life: perspectives of people with mental illnesses and family members. Psychiatr Rehabil J 25:350–359, 2002

26. Johnson ED: Differences among families coping with serious mental illness: a qualitative analysis. Am J Orthopsychiatry 70:126–134, 2000

27. Boyce P: Restoring wisdom to the practice of psychiatry. Australas Psychiatry 14:3–7, 2006

8

Family/Couples Therapy: Models

- Many schools or models of family treatment exist.
- Choose one or two models to learn well.

There are many competing models of understanding and treating family disorders, each with its unique mediating and final goals; these are reviewed and compared in this chapter. This review of models is not comprehensive or exhaustive. The goal is to recognize that there are many different ways in which interpersonal and family issues can be conceptualized and potentially changed. Clinicians have to decide for themselves which approach fits best with their worldview, personality style, and therapeutic capabilities.

An observer of the general psychotherapy field has stated (1):

> In picking up the textbook of the future, we should see in the table of contents not a listing of School A, School B, and so on—perhaps ending with the author's attempt at integration—but an outline of the various agreed-upon intervention principles, a specification of varying techniques for implementing each principle, and an indication of the relative effectiveness of each of these techniques, together with their interaction with varying presenting problems and individual differences among patients/clients and therapists.

Unfortunately, even three decades later, there is insufficient evidence to compile such a table of contents with any degree of objectivity. Many couples/ family therapy models have not been rigorously tested with different patient/ client populations and have rarely been compared with each other. Dismantling studies designed to try to understand the active ingredients of the different schools have also not been carried out. Few studies have been under-taken to match patient characteristics or deficits to particular therapeutic ap-proaches. None of this means that the various therapeutic approaches do not work but rather that we cannot say one works better than another for a par-ticular population. It is important to be aware of and to have some familiarity with a variety of ways of understanding and helping families because all mod-els provide some useful perspectives. Ultimately, however, we believe it is most useful from a clinical perspective to become skilled in one or two. We present in this chapter the general schools or models of family intervention by focus-ing not primarily on their originators but on their mediating and final goals and related strategies of intervention.

Much has been written about the diverse schools of family intervention, often formed around the so-called first and second generation of charismatic leaders. There are different classifications of the schools, each with their own assumptions about the origin and maintenance of pathology, goals, strategies, and techniques for intervention and indications for utilization. It is useful for the student of family interventions to have some conceptual understanding of these schools, their history, and the contemporary personalities involved (see Table 8–1).

Insight Awareness Model

The insight awareness orientation has also been known as the historical, psy-chodynamic, or psychoanalytic school. In a real sense, this is the oldest school of family therapy because it grew out of the psychoanalytic tradition.

By changing transference distortions, correcting projective identifica-tions, and infusing insight and new understanding into the area of interper-sonal turmoil and conflict, this school of family therapy attempts to change the functioning and interrelationships of the various members of the family or marital system. Information about the family is derived from historical ma-terial of the current and past generations, transference/countertransference phenomena, unconscious derivatives, and resistances. A basic assumption is that intrapsychic conflict, interpersonal problem foci, and defensive and cop-ing mechanisms are modeled and played out within the family system. Dream and fantasy material, fantasies and projections about other family members, and transference distortions about other family members and the therapist are of paramount interest to these practitioners. Understanding the history and mutations over time of these dynamics is considered crucial to understanding current dysfunction.

A broad use of the terms *transference* and *countertransference* is applied here. These phenomena can be understood in at least five directions: 1) man to woman, 2) woman to man, 3) woman to therapist, 4) man to therapist, and 5) couple (or family) to therapist. (Note that "man" and "woman" can refer to either therapist or client.) Just as there are multiple transference reactions, there are multiple countertransference responses. It is assumed that understanding unconscious derivatives and their resistances is necessary to effect change.

The theoretical underpinnings of this model are the familiar ones of psychoanalytic thinking, such as topographical concepts of conscious, preconscious, and unconscious constructs of the id, ego, and superego, as well as concepts that focus on the interaction of individuals, such as secondary gain, transference, and projective identification. While early analysts who opted for a more interactional model criticized this model for its lack of attention to, and language for, interactional data, others in the analytic tradition of object relations have applied these concepts to the understanding and analytic treatment of these interactional problems.

The major therapeutic techniques of this model include clarification, interpretation, exploration of intrapsychic as well as interpersonal dynamics, and development of insight and empathy. Using analytic techniques with an individual in the presence of a spouse or other family member represented a unique development in its time. However, more important is the understanding of current mutual distortions and projections in the couple's interaction. The goal is to foster understanding and insight to effect change in both individuals and the family unit.

Family-of-Origin Model

Allied with the psychodynamic model is the family-of-origin model, which uses historical data as key. This group of theorists is most interested in the realities of the three- and four-generation family—its themes, beliefs, loyalties from past generations, and the immediate functioning of adult patients and their parents rather than patient fantasies about them. In this model the

Table 8–1. Models of family treatment

Treatment approach ("school")	Representative therapies	Strategies and techniques	Stance	Goals	Database
1. Insight-awareness (also known as historical, psychodynamic, or psychoanalytic)	Ackerman Borzormenyi-Nagy and Spark Paul Nadelson Bowen (2)	1. Observation 2. Clarification 3. Interpretation	1. Listener 2. "Therapeutic distance" 3. Therapeutic stance of technical neutrality	Foster understanding and insight to effect change	1. History 2. Unconscious derivatives 3. Transference
2. Systemic strategic (also known as systems, communications, or structural)	Palo Alto Group (Jackson, Bateson, Haley, Satir) Sluzki Bowen (2) Minuchin (8) M. Erickson Palazzoli	1. Strategies to alter family structure and behavior 2. Observe and transform using directives	Therapist observes and moves in and out of process	Change structure, communication pattern, and roles, which change perception and behavior	1. Sequences 2. Communication 3. Rules 4. History
3. Cognitive-behavioral	R. Weiss Jacobson (10) Patterson I. Falloon Epstein (11)	1. Communication teaching 2. Problem-solving skills 3. Contingency contracting	Therapist is collaborator in the development of interpersonal skills	Eliminate dysfunctional behaviors and learn to utilize new and more effective interpersonal behaviors	1. Observation of overt behaviors 2. Functional analysis of problematic behavioral sequences

Table 8–1. Models of family treatment (*continued*)

Treatment approach ("school")	Representative therapies	Strategies and techniques	Stance	Goals	Database
4. Experiential-existential	Napier and Whitaker (12) Bowen (2) Borzormenyi-Nagy (4) Satir (6)	1. Therapist designs and/or participates with family in the emotional experience 2. Empathy	Therapist offers self for interaction to minimize distance between family and self	1. Change ways family members experience (and presumably react to) each other 2. Growth and differentiation	1. Observed verbal and nonverbal behavior 2. Shared feelings (including the therapist's feelings)
5. Narrative	White and Epston (9)	1. Externalizing the problem 2. Mapping influence of problem over family and influence of family over the problem	Therapist collaborates with family on a therapeutic conversation	1. Develop an alternative narrative story about the problem 2. Liberate the family from being controlled by the problem toward authoring their own study	Linguistic behavior

spouses are encouraged and coached to deal with their issues directly with members of the family of origin so as not to project them onto their spouses. In the main, this model encourages understanding of the parents and individuation within the family rather than confrontation.

Each of these family theorists is identified with a different model within the broad range of interest in looking at three-generational families. Bowen (2) developed family systems theory in which he focused on the role of the family's emotional system in the etiology of individual dysfunction. His theory concentrated on the need to differentiate oneself within the family by distinguishing between intellectual process and the feeling the person is experiencing; he focused on family triangles, the family projection process, and multigenerational transmission. Bowen's therapy works with individuals, coaching them how to differentiate within the family.

Framo (3) is usually grouped with object relations therapists. While others are more interested in seeing the whole family of origin together and concentrating on reconnection, Framo's model starts with the couple, but each spouse separately explores relationships with all family members. Framo also developed a model of working with couples groups. Borzormenyi-Nagy and Krasner (4) developed contextual therapy, which emphasizes loyalty, balance, and relational justice. Williamson (5), Framo, and Borzormenyi-Nagy and Krasner all work with multigenerational families in the therapy room. Advantages to this model include its emphasis on personal and family growth, rather than pathology, and its inherent commonsense appeal to many people.

Systemic Strategic Model

As systems theory developed, a variety of therapists decided to push the envelope to see how far they could take a therapy in which the only emphasis was on the here-and-now system and current relationships (6). In these models, it was assumed that the individual is governed and regulated by the system and that changing the repetitive patterns of communication and behavior between them in the present would eliminate symptomatology. A variety of models were proposed for symptom production, including the idea that the symptom was needed for the homeostasis of the system, or that the family's efforts to solve the problem had led to more problems (the solution becoming the problem). The ultimate goal of therapy is to change the pattern. Insight or understanding is not a goal of treatment, although often it occurs as a result. In these models it is considered the job of the therapist to understand the problem and find a solution, as opposed to models, which are more collaborative.

Treatment techniques include focusing on, exaggerating, deemphasizing, or relabeling symptoms; clarifying communication; interrupting repetitive interactional patterns; or prescribing symptoms. For example, a family may come in with the complaint that the daughter does not obey the mother and is becoming impossible to discipline. If the father and daughter look at each other and smile whenever the mother attempts to make a statement, the therapist could ask the mother and daughter to speak directly to each other and ask the father to support the mother. The therapist could also exaggerate the problem by telling the father that every time the girl disobeys her mother, he should congratulate her or give her a dime. This would bring the problem out in the open and force the father to disown his covert support of the girl's behavior. Alternatively, the therapist could label the daughter's behavior as spoiled instead of psychiatrically troubled and inquire why the father was letting his daughter behave in this way. None of these interventions require history or insight. It is important to emphasize that systems theory (like the other models) has limitations depending on the problems of any particular family (7).

Structural Model

The structural model, pioneered by Minuchin and Fishman (8), is probably the most known and most used of the systems theories. It is less focused on details of communication and more on the family "dance" or structure. Minuchin is particularly interested in hierarchy (parental subsystems should be in charge of child subsystems) and clear boundaries, so that each member has a sense of self and privacy but also a sense of "familyness." It is important to understand, however, that boundaries, hierarchies, and coalitions are repetitive behaviors (both verbal and nonverbal) determined by the operational rules and beliefs of the family. These patterns arrange or organize the family's function. The structural model is particularly good at setting up situations in which the new structure is modeled in session (e.g., "Mom, you and dad sit next to each other and decide how to handle this problem with your child"), as well as giving tasks to continue the structure at home.

The models of systems theory in which present-oriented and family-focused techniques are used exclusively have been modified extensively over the last 20 years. Most practitioners see the system as composed of subsystems that must be understood, including the biological system of each individual and the internal myths, stories, and beliefs by which each individual modifies incoming communications. Most therapists today are interested in how a person's story of his or her past affects present behavior, and they use this knowledge in reframing the current situation or in developing directives. This has been referred to as the narrative model (9).

Cognitive-Behavioral Model

The behavioral model grew out of the behavioral orientation that has historically flourished parallel with and in reaction to the psychoanalytic tradition. The data for this orientation are quantifiable, measurable behaviors, whether internal (thoughts) or external (actions) (10). Explanatory concepts are derived from learning theories, for example, concepts such as stimulus, response, classical conditioning, operant conditioning, and schedules of reinforcement. With the behavioral model becoming increasingly applied to interactional systems such as the family, other concepts have been introduced to expand the model into the interpersonal sphere. Perhaps the most influential theory has been the behavior exchange model, in which it is postulated that there is a benefit and cost ratio for each individual in an exchange situation (e.g., marriage). What that ratio is has a major influence on the course and outcome of that relationship. For example, if one spouse receives (what is perceived as) only a little benefit in exchange for a lot of effort, it would increase the risk of the marriage failing.

The goal in the cognitive-behavioral model is to effect change in discrete, observable, measurable behaviors that are considered problematic by the individuals seeking assistance (11). As opposed to the psychoanalytic model, which often seems to have more ambitious goals of character change and insight, this model focuses more on discrete problem areas defined by clear behavior patterns. Thus, treatment in this model tends to be briefer and more circumscribed. Emphasis is placed not on pathology but on behavioral deficits and excesses that are to be changed. If undesired behaviors are eliminated (e.g., intimate partner violence), it is not assumed that more social behaviors will necessarily spontaneously emerge, but rather that the therapist may be required to teach new and more adaptive behaviors to the spouses or family members.

Techniques include helping family members learn how to elicit the desired behavior in another member. Some of the major tactics include behavioral contracting based on good faith or quid pro quo agreements ("If you do this, I will do that"), training in communication skills, training in effective problem solving, and combining positive reinforcement with a decrease in destructive interchanges. In the last several years cognitive issues have been given more attention, especially the meaning of behavior ("Is he doing it because he loves me or because he is forced to?") and the cognitions behind behavioral choice ("I must not say I am sorry, even though I am, because it makes me feel less of a man"). This model has also been more willing to focus on the gender problems that make negotiating more difficult—for example, can the couple really negotiate, as equals, a mutually acceptable agreement on behavior when the husband earns a million dollars a year and the wife has no skills or training and believes she cannot leave the marriage? This inherent inequity makes change more difficult.

The stance of the therapist is actively to introduce behavior change into the repertoire of the family members. Although behaviorists have written less about how they handle individual and family resistance to suggestions, the increased focus on cognitions and meanings is beginning to shift, with recent writings focusing more on systemic interventions such as reversals or restraint of change.

This school of family therapy in general does not concentrate on eliciting much historical material, expressing buried feelings, or interpreting psychodynamics. Understanding and insight are much less important in producing change. Active suggestion, direction, and homework are its hallmarks.

Although the majority of family therapists would not call themselves cognitive-behavioral therapists, these techniques have been used to some extent by almost all therapists at one time or another. The goal is to change the way family members experience and presumably react to each other. A secondary goal is growth and differentiation of family members.

Experiential Models

Experiential therapy involves a search for meaning through mutually shared experience on the part of the therapist and family. Carl Whitaker (12) and Virginia Satir (6) were two of the best-known therapists of this model. Both had as a goal the idea of increasing the family members' capacity to experience their lives more fully by sharing with the therapist the struggle with the here and now.

Whitaker's work, called *symbolic experiential therapy*, aimed to strengthen the unconscious symbolic processes that foster maturation. This approach emphasizes the therapist's participation as a whole person rather than as an interpreter or director in the process. Assumptions of this model are that growth in families occurs spontaneously and occurs with the mastery of successive developmental tasks. Prior sets of assumptions must be dissolved before new assumptions can replace them. Therapy works to catalyze this process rather than impose a predetermined structure. Symptoms are regarded as frustrated attempts at growth. Symptom removal is not the primary goal of therapy but is considered the byproduct. Integration of the "split-off" aspects of the family's experience is the main objective. The therapist uses both technical skills/ knowledge and nonrational responses (intuitions, fantasies, dreams, affect), which affect the family at a powerful affective level and evoke their latent symbolic conflicts. In Whitaker's model, the assumption is that if the family disorganizes by talking about usually hidden things, it will relinquish its logical defensive structures and then reorganize in more constructive ways. His model, intuitive and idiosyncratic, is difficult to teach but thought to be powerful in practice.

Satir's model operates less in the fantasy dimension and more in the here and now. These models remind us that structure and problem solving are not the only possible goals of family therapy but that a warm and connected listener who is open to deeper structures and meanings has much to offer.

Constructivist Model

Among the newer additions to the field of family therapy is a set of assumptions falling loosely under the rubric "constructivism," part of what has been called the postmodern movement in philosophy and psychology. It is based on the work of a series of theorists from epistemology, biology, and cybernetics who see reality as constructed by the observer rather than as an objective truth to be discovered. Translated into the field of therapy, this suggests that the *family's reality* is in its shared narratives and meaning systems, that the *personal story* or *self-narrative* provides the principal frame of intelligibility for people's lived experience, and that the therapist's assumptions about the family are also constructed rather than "truth." The job of the therapist, then, is to help the family explore and reevaluate its own assumptions, beliefs, and meaning systems. In this model, a dysfunctional family has constructed a series of meanings that are not working and thus are preventing the family from being flexible and functioning well. For example, if the mother is defined as "bad," any move she makes toward either comforting or disciplining will be ignored, which means the children get neither comfort nor discipline. If her story is constructed differently by the family, for example, as "mother is doing her best to function in spite of her difficulties," she will be able to take care of the family because they will accept her care. This model allows therapist and patient together to *deconstruct* confining family stories, which produce stasis or sadness, and to consider new ones. Rather than the therapist producing a reframe and convincing the family of its correctness, the constructivist model emphasizes the importance of collaboration and mutual respect in the therapeutic alliance. Treatment is primarily conceptualized as a conversation about problems in which new meanings and new behaviors can be considered. Unlike schools that highlight the family's history or structural organization, these approaches highlight the strengths and competencies of the family that are often occluded by the family's and therapist's tendency to focus on the specific problems that bring the family to treatment.

Different therapists have used these ideas in different ways to address family problems. The solution-oriented approach has been championed by Steve deShazer (13) and Bill O'Hanlon (14). Its aims are to build on the growth-enhancing part of people's lives. The model focuses on specific solutions to problems rather than on personal growth, and it helps the client create new stories by focusing on "exceptions"—times when the problem did not occur. This allows for the development of new and more competent stories.

Michael White and his colleagues in Australia (9) have developed a model of externalizing problems so that "the problem" becomes a separate entity, external to the person who has it. This allows for a move away from a problem-saturated story about the person himself or herself to a person or group of people working together defeating it. One might, for example, ask, "How is 'bulimia' working to keep you from your friends?" In both approaches, problems are viewed as oppressively intruding on people's abilities to lead more fulfilling lives. At the same time, these problems are also seen as unacknowledged insidious extensions of both historical and sociocultural influences (e.g., inequities related to gender, race, class, ethnicity, or sexual orientation).

In some ways the constructivist position has returned psychiatry to its roots, by elevating meaning to a position at least equal in importance to behavior patterns and by increasing attention to one's own meaning and value systems. Discussion continues over whether relativism can be taken too far and whether any solution acceptable to the family is acceptable to the therapist.

Psychoeducational Model

The psychoeducational model is most commonly used in conjunction with psychiatric disorders, less so with problems and life-change issues. It is defined as the systematic administration of information to both patient and family (significant others) about signs and symptoms, diagnosis, treatment, and prognosis. Its aim is behavioral change and not just teaching for the sake of increasing knowledge. It must be given in "doses," as the recipients are "able to hear it," and given repetitively over time.

Multifamily Group Therapy

The multifamily group therapy model combines elements from family therapy and group therapy in a psychoeducational context. Although it often requires a cotherapist, this model is still relatively cost-effective because it brings a number of families together at the same time.

The major stages in the treatment program for multifamily groups are joining with individual patients and families, conducting educational workshops for families, preventing relapse through the use of problem-solving groups attended by both patients and families, and encouraging vocational and social rehabilitation (15). The general goals of these groups are to help patients and family members become knowledgeable about the signs and symptoms of the illness. The group increases the members' understanding of the effects of the illness by sharing information, support, and its members' own perspectives on family interactions. Patients and family members gain insight and learn new coping strategies in dealing with different phases of the patient's illness. Patients and families develop a better understanding of how they can work with each other and with mental health professionals to deal with a difficult and chronic illness. This model balances educational information about the illness with guided discussions in which patients and family members share their personal experiences and concerns in coping with the illness. Information on operationalizing the logistics of organizing and conducting such a group is readily available (16).

Conclusion

Currently there are many strategies for treating families. Each may emphasize different assumptions and types of interventions. Some therapists prefer to operate with one strategy in most cases, whereas others mix these strategies depending on the type of case and the phase of treatment. At times the strategy used is made explicit by the therapist, whereas in other instances it remains covert. Irrespective of whether a therapist specializes in one or another approach or is eclectic, some hypotheses will be formed about the nature of the family's difficulty and the preferred approach.

With the therapeutic focus on one person, the emphasis is often on the individual's perceptions, reactions, and feelings, and also on the equality of status between the individual and the therapist. When two people are the operative system, attention is directed to interactions and relationships. Therapists who think in terms of a unit of three people look at coalitions, structures, and hierarchies of status and power. The number of people actually involved in the interviews may not be as important as how many people are involved in the therapist's way of thinking about the problem.

Some therapists emphasize reconstruction of past events, whereas others choose to deal only with current behavior as manifested during the therapy session. Some therapists favor verbal exploration and interpretation, whereas others favor using an action or experiential mode of treatment, either in the session itself or by requiring new behavior outside the interview. Some therapists think in terms of problems and symptoms and attempt to decode or understand possible symbolic meanings of symptomatology, whereas other therapists focus on the potentials for growth and differentiation that are not being fulfilled. Some therapists utilize one or a very limited number of methods in dealing with a whole range of problems, whereas others are more eclectic and attempt to tailor the treatment techniques to what they consider the specific requirements of the situation.

Therapists may choose one school or another based on their training or their personality. For example, a very organized and directive person would probably prefer cognitive-behavioral methods, whereas a person who prefers long-term emotional intensity over problem solving might gravitate to experiential models. Individuals and families as well may prefer certain ways of working over others. It is difficult for therapists to become proficient in many therapy models. There is a risk of becoming superficial, facile, and inconsistent, leaving families uneasy about the lack of direction and focus in therapy. Therapeutic tools from different schools may be useful, but a skilled couples/family therapist is likely to use one or two conceptual frameworks to guide his or her treatment.

References

1. Goldfried M: Toward the delineation of therapeutic change principles. Am Psychol 35:997–998, 1980
2. Bowen M: Family Therapy in Clinical Practice. New York, Aronson, 1978
3. Framo JL: Family-of-Origin Therapy: An Intergenerational Approach. New York, Brunner/Mazel, 1992
4. Borzormenyi-Nagy I, Krasner B: Give and Take: A Clinical Guide to Contextual Therapy. New York, Brunner/Mazel, 1986
5. Williamson D: The Intimacy Paradox: Personal Authority in the Family System. New York, Guilford, 1986
6. Satir V: Conjoint Family Therapy: A Guide to Theory and Technique. Palo Alto, CA, Science and Behavior Books, 1964
7. Merkel WT, Searight HR: Why families are not like swamps, solar systems, or thermostats: some limits of systems theory as applied to family therapy. Contemporary Family Therapy 14:33–50, 1992
8. Minuchin S, Fishman HC: Family Therapy Techniques. Cambridge, MA, Harvard University Press, 1981
9. White M, Epston D: Narrative Means to Therapeutic Ends. New York, WW Norton, 1990

10. Jacobson NS, Margolin G: Marital Therapy. New York, Brunner/Mazel, 1979
11. Ryan CE, Epstein N, Keitner GI, et al: Evaluating and Treating Families: The McMaster Approach. New York, Routledge Taylor & Francis Group, 2005
12. Napier AY, Whitaker CA: The Family Crucible. New York, Harper & Row, 1978
13. deShazer S: Investigating Solutions in Brief Therapy. New York, WW Norton, 1988
14. O'Hanlon WH, Weiner-Davis M: In Search of Solutions: A New Direction in Psychotherapy. New York, WW Norton, 1989
15. McFarlane WR: Multifamily Groups in the Treatment of Severe Psychiatric Disorders. New York, Guilford, 2002
16. Keitner GI, Drury LM, Ryan CE, et al: Multifamily group treatment for major depressive disorder, in Multifamily Groups in the Treatment of Severe Psychiatric Disorders. Edited by McFarlane WR. New York, Guilford, 2002, pp 244–267

Suggested Readings

Gurman A, Kniskern D, eds: Handbook of Family Therapy, Vol. I and II. New York, Brunner/Mazel, 1981   [This edited volume provides an excellent introduction to the major models of family therapy. The book is well organized, and chapters are written by noted representatives of each of the influential schools.]

Lebow J: The integrative revolution in couple and family therapy. Fam Process 36:1–19, 1997   [This article examines the present status of integrative models of therapy, including specific conceptual developments and directions. The author demonstrates the direction in which the field is headed.]

9

Problem-Centered Systems Therapy of the Family

- Problem-Centered Systems Therapy of the Family (PCSTF) is the therapeutic component of a comprehensive model (the McMaster Model) of family functioning.
- PCSTF is a problem-focused and behaviorally directed therapy that empowers families to work more effectively together.
- PCSTF focuses on stages of treatment rather than on specific intervention skills or the particular personality style of the therapist.
- PCSTF is manualized, allowing for easier learning and consistent application.
- PCSTF has been empirically validated as being useful in the management of a number of disorders.

There are many schools of family therapy just as there are many schools of individual psychotherapy. A number of these models of family therapies are reviewed in Chapter 8. In general, there is no empirical evidence to suggest that one form of family therapy is more effective than another, although some forms have been more systematically tested for particular psychiatric disorders, as outlined in Chapter 3.

The lack of evidence about the relative effectiveness of different forms of family therapy leads to a dilemma for a clinician trying to determine which family approach to learn and which one to use in particular clinical situations. This dilemma may lead to two opposite attempts at resolution. One extreme resolution may be to become too rigidly committed to a narrow approach in dealing with families. The other extreme is to try to become familiar with and learn a wide variety of family approaches to pick and choose those aspects of different schools of family therapy that may seem applicable to a given clinical situation. The first approach carries the risk that the therapist may become too narrow, rigid, and dogmatic, thereby missing the opportunity to be more broadly effective in dealing with family problems. The second approach carries the risk of conceptual confusion, diffusion of focus, and practical inconsistencies, all of which may aggravate the uncertainty and chaos that often characterizes problems presented by families in distress.

It is more advantageous for a therapist to become competent in one major school of family therapy and familiar with a few others to be able to undertake family therapy in a clear and consistent way. Therapists need to be aware of models that allow for different perspectives on a wide range of presenting problems. It is difficult enough to become skilled in one form of family therapy. Attempting to be a master of all may well lead to being a master of none. It is important to learn a model of family therapy that is broadly based and well defined so as to allow it to be applied to a wide range of family problems. The Problem-Centered Systems Therapy of the Family (PCSTF) is one such model (1). It is a problem-focused, behaviorally directed family therapy model that empowers families to work effectively on resolving their distressing situation.

There are a number of compelling reasons why the PCSTF may be a useful model to learn as the foundation for dealing with families. It is based on the McMaster Model of Family Functioning (2), which describes and assesses normative functioning along a broad range of family dimensions. Instead of focusing on only a few areas of family functioning such as communications and problems solving, the McMaster Model helps the therapist evaluate and help the family to resolve issues in a number of additional aspects of family life, including the way that they connect with each other, allocate roles, set standards of behavior, and deal with each other's emotional responsivity (see Chapter 4). The treatment approach has been spelled out in a manual, thus allowing for easier learning and dissemination. The PCSTF also has assessment instruments (the Family Assessment Device and the Clinical Rating Scale) that allow for systematic and quantifiable evaluation of family functions from both the families' and an external rater's perspective. These evaluations can be used for both research purposes and tracking clinical changes in family functioning over time as treatment progresses.

PCSTF: basic principles

- Importance of a comprehensive assessment
- Inclusion of as many family members as possible
- Emphasis on macro stages of treatment
- Therapist modeling of open and direct communication with the family
- Active collaboration with the family
- Focus on family's strengths
- Family responsibility for change
- Focus on current problems
- Emphasis on behavioral change
- Short term and time limited

A unique feature of the PCSTF is that it focuses on stages of treatment rather than on specific intervention skills or particular personality characteristics of the therapist. These stages are referred to as the macro stages of treatment and differ from micro family techniques, which occur within the macro stages. The PCSTF is also relatively free of culturally laden value assumptions.

The major value attached to the model is that optimal family functioning is most likely to be achieved when there is open, direct, and clear communication between family members. Apart from this expectation, the model leaves it up to the family to determine which aspects of their family's lives they are content with and which they wish to see change regardless of how an external evaluator may see the family's problems. The only exception to this rule is when there is evidence of dangerous behavior in the family, such as physical or emotional abuse of any family members. These principles are summarized below. Finally, the PCSTF has been empirically validated as a useful adjunct in the treatment of patients with mood disorders (see Chapter 3).

Key Principles of PCSTF

Importance of a Comprehensive Assessment

PCSTF emphasizes the need for a comprehensive understanding of the family system, including its problems and strengths, as fully as possible. In addition to the presenting problems, the assessment includes understanding the structure, organization, and transactional patterns within the family. The assessment process includes reviewing multiple dimensions of family life as described in Chapter 4. Similar to a mental status examination, the family's ways of communicating, solving problems, experiencing emotional connectedness, dealing with emotions, allocating roles, and setting standards within the family need to be reviewed. The presenting problem may not necessarily be the most important one. Focusing prematurely on the presenting problem without understanding the broader context in which it plays out may lead to a preoccupation with peripheral issues and missing a problem that may be generating the most distress.

In uncomplicated cases, a thorough assessment that clearly defines the family's problems is therapeutic. Many such families are able to then proceed to deal with their problems without further treatment. In families with more complicated problems, however, a comprehensive assessment can clearly delineate the various components that need to be addressed to develop the most effective treatment plan. A thorough assessment also reassures the family members that they are being understood and helps them to take a step back to understand their problems from a broader perspective. When dealing with a family emergency, the therapist needs to be active and focused. The immediate issue needs to be dealt with (e.g., hospitalization for suicidality, restraining order for spousal abuse), after which a more comprehensive family assessment can still take place.

Inclusion of the Entire Family

It is preferable to include as many family members as possible, at least for the initial assessment. Having all family members present (including extended family or close friends) facilitates obtaining a full range of views, an understanding of potential support systems, and direct observation of parent, child, and sibling interactions. Having all family members present also gives a clear signal that everybody is involved in the process and that each person may have an impact on outcome.

Such an open and collaborative meeting can also encourage family members to participate actively in the treatment process. Another reason for including as many family members as possible is that in many families there is often one family member who is carrying a disproportionate burden of the family's problems. If appropriately supported, this person can be very helpful in outlining the true nature of the family's issues. In each family a different person may carry this role. By having all family members present, there is a greater chance of including this person in the treatment process.

In the course of treatment it may be necessary to limit the participants, depending on issues being discussed (e.g., sexuality) or logistics concerning the ability of various family members to participate in the available time. In general, however, the larger number of family members that can participate, the more likely there is to be a satisfactory outcome. Some family members are concerned about involving others in their problems on the assumption that it may make the situation worse by highlighting problems of which others may not have been aware. In general, however, there are few long-standing family problems that those living together are not aware of or affected by. Most family members are usually relieved to know that the family is receiving professional help, that the professional involved is trying to address difficulties they may be experiencing, and that there is opportunity for resolution to the problematic situation.

Emphasis on Macro Stages of Treatment

Macro stages refer to the major stages of treatment. These stages are assessment, contracting, treatment, and closure. Therapists make use of a variety of strategies and interventions as a way of leading a family through the macro stages. The macro stages and the strategies required to navigate families through them are different from micro moves, which are specific interviewing and intervention skills (3). Micro moves include such techniques as labeling, focusing the family on a particular problem, and clarifying communication patterns.

The macro stages and the micro moves are different from a therapist's particular personality style, which may include qualities such as choice of wording, use of gestures, and ways of helping families look at difficult situations. A number of family therapy schools have become well known because of the particular personality style and skills of a charismatic family therapist. Not surprisingly, a family therapy model that depends on such individual and unique personal qualities is very difficult to teach and replicate. The PCSTF focuses on the stages and steps in therapy and depends less on the particular personality of the therapist. The PCSTF accommodates therapists with a variety of clinical styles.

Therapists may also vary in their repertoire and skill in utilizing micro interventions such as focusing the family or labeling process. Understandably, the more skill that a therapist has in applying a wider range of micro moves, the more likely he or she will be efficient in carrying out family treatment. Expert therapists are likely to use a broader range of skills and advanced techniques when applying the PCSTF model. Less experienced therapists will use the PCSTF as a basis for a structured treatment approach while developing more tactical skills. Nonetheless, if the steps and sequences defined in the therapy approach are adhered to, most therapists, including beginning therapists, can be reasonably effective in working with the majority of families who present with problems. The PCSTF posits that the most likely ingredient for bringing about effective change is the process of leading the family through the macro stages of therapy.

Therapist Modeling of Open and Direct Communication With the Family

The therapist explains his or her formulations and actions in an open and direct way with the family at each step of the therapy process and makes sure the family members clearly understand and agree along the way. This openness fosters collaboration and empowers the family to feel they can play a significant role in bringing about change within themselves. By being open and direct, the therapist also models for the family an effective way of dealing with problems. In general, the PCSTF underplays the importance of indirect or paradoxical interventions. The PCSTF assumes that family members understand their problems and are interested in changing them and that they have the capacity to do so with support and guidance.

Active Collaboration With the Family

The PCSTF stresses active collaboration with the family at each stage of the treatment process. Active collaboration with all family members reinforces the therapeutic alliance between the therapist and the family. The family needs to be an active and willing participant in each step of the treatment. There needs to be agreement between the therapist and family members, both about the formulation of the presenting problem and about the steps that are likely to be helpful in resolving them. The family also has to be committed to following through on the steps agreed upon to bring about the desired change in the family. The therapeutic contract is based on this mutual commitment to work at therapy.

Focus on Family's Strengths

The PCSTF explicitly recognizes that all families have strengths that should be recognized and fostered during treatment. It is much easier and more helpful to the family to reinforce its strengths rather than trying to eliminate its weaknesses. Too much focus on pathology begets pathology. Given that a core feature of the model is its emphasis on the family's capacity and responsibility for change, it is important that the therapist help the family to recognize its own capacities to address and deal with difficult situations.

Family's Responsibility for Change

The PCSTF makes clear to the family members that they will be doing most of the therapy work. Family members are directly involved in identifying, clarifying, and resolving the difficulties and problems of the family. The role of the therapist is that of a catalyst, clarifier, and facilitator. The therapist helps the family to be more open with each other, to communicate more clearly with each other, and to be active in their problem solving. The goal is to have family members become more aware of their strengths as well as their shortcomings and to develop effective problem-solving methods that can be generalized to resolve future difficulties. By working actively on current problems, they learn the skills needed to deal with problems that may crop up in the future.

Focus on Current Problems

The PCSTF focuses largely on current problems. During the assessment process and when appropriate during the course of treatment, it may be necessary to review past issues to obtain a full understanding of how the current problem came about, what it means to individual family members, and what attempts have been made at resolution. In general, however, once the evolution and meaning of the problem is understood, the focus is on what the family wants to do about it now.

Emphasis on Behavioral Change

Changing attitudes, beliefs, and opinions are important, but the PCSTF emphasizes change primarily in observable behaviors. Such changes in behavior are the defined goals of treatment. This focus on behaviors does not deny the importance of cognitions or affect but recognizes that behavioral change is most manifest and measurable. Changes in behavior could lead to changes in cognitions and affect as much as changes in cognitions and affect may lead to changes in behavior. It is much easier to change what one does than what one thinks and feels.

Short Term and Time Limited

The PCSTF is, in general, a short-term time-limited treatment, taking on average 6–12 sessions spaced over a period of weeks, months, or a year. The length of each individual session or the time between them will vary depending on the issues involved, the stage of treatment, and the urgency of the situation. The early assessment session(s) may take longer and be spaced more closely to ensure a quick but comprehensive understanding of the problem, whereas later task-setting treatment sessions may be as short as 15 to 20 minutes.

In the assessment and early treatment sessions, the family can be seen weekly. If all goes well, treatment sessions are then likely to be spread out to every 2 weeks, then once a month, and then, if still needed, additional follow-up every 3–6 months. In between sessions, the family is expected to work on the identified problems and tasks that were agreed on during the treatment sessions.

The PCSTF tries to limit the number of treatment sessions for a number of reasons. Imposing time limitations on therapy sessions tends to stimulate therapists and families to be more actively involved in the treatment process, thereby facilitating change. Without set time limits, therapists and families often develop a mutually satisfying but not necessarily effective relationship. Defining a limited number of sessions communicates to the family that the therapist is confident in the family's ability to work at effecting change. More complicated family situations and those families dealing with chronic relapsing and remitting illnesses may need to be seen for a longer period of time. If treatment does persist beyond 12 sessions, reevaluation of the treatment situation, and possibly consultation, should be considered.

An example of the early stage of treatment is presented in the DVD accompanying this manual. The assessment of the family is described in the appendix to Chapter 4. The appendix to this present chapter reviews one aspect of the treatment contract and shows what to do when the family members are successful in accomplishing their goals and what to do when they are not.

Stages of Treatment

The four macro stages of treatment

- Assessment
- Contracting
- Treatment
- Closure

The four macro stages of treatment comprising the PCSTF are assessment, contracting, treatment, and closure. Each stage contains a sequence of substages, the first of which is always orientation.

Orientation at each stage of the process is a critical component of the therapeutic process. From the initial encounter, family members need to be oriented as to what to expect. Their agreement and permission to proceed need to be obtained before treatment can begin. Directness and clarity of purpose not only eliminate potential misunderstandings in terms of expectations and assumptions but also model a way of approaching potentially difficult situations. They show respect for the family, empower the family in preparation for therapeutic work, and strengthen the therapeutic alliance. Orientation to the assessment stage is the most detailed and sets the tone and direction for the therapy to come. Orientation to the later stages of treatment may be briefer and more specific to the particular focus and tasks at hand at that point in time. Orientation is a time to set explicit rules and expectations for the treatment process. The family's agreement with the goals outlined can be useful in minimizing resistance that may emerge in later stages, reminding families of their agreement to collaborate in the treatment goals.

Assessment

Substages of assessment

- Orientation
- Data gathering
- Problem description
- Problem clarification

The assessment stage is made up of the following substages: orientation, data gathering, problem description, and problem clarification. The assessment stage is clearly the most important of the macro stages of the PCSTF. As emphasized throughout this book, the first step in effective treatment is the development of a comprehensive and meaningful biopsychosocial formulation of the problem(s). The assessment stage is the time during which information and observations are gathered so as to be able to develop this formulation.

The assessment stage has three main goals. First, the therapist orients the family to the treatment process and establishes an open collaborative relationship with family members. Second, the therapist, with the help of family members, identifies all current problems in the family, including the presenting problem. Third, the therapist identifies the family's dynamic interactional patterns that appear to be related to the family's problems. The issues that the therapist has formulated are presented to the family for acceptance as accurate or for revision as needed.

Because of the importance of the assessment, the therapist should take as many sessions as necessary to complete it. The number of assessment sessions required will vary depending on the therapist's expertise and the extent and nature of the family's problems. In general, the extra time taken in the assessment stage will reduce the number of task-oriented treatment sessions that will be required later in the treatment process. The process of identifying, clarifying, and understanding various family members' perspectives of the problems at hand are often therapeutic in and of themselves.

It is important to maintain the interest of and connection with families during a protracted assessment process. If the assessment is going to take more than a few sessions, it is important to summarize findings at the end of each session up to that point, listen carefully to the family's reaction to the summary, and clarify what additional information is being sought. Assessment sessions should not be spaced more than a week apart. Families presenting for help are looking for feedback and an outside perspective on their situation as well as a sense of what can be done within a defined time frame. If some feedback is not provided quickly, families will become frustrated and drop out of treatment. Information about what the therapist has noticed to date and likely further steps can be provided without coming to a premature closure of the assessment process and without setting up false expectations.

The assessment is based on family members' reports of their perception of the situation. The therapist confirms his or her impressions of the issues reported by family members by observing the family's behavior during the assessment process. A more comprehensive evaluation can also occur when a therapist tries to clarify contradictions between information gathered from different members or contradictions between their descriptions of family functioning and the interpersonal processes observed by the therapist during the assessment session. In addition to clarifying the issues at hand, highlighting discrepancies also models for the family a way of resolving differences between family members' perspectives that is nonthreatening and supportive of the overall goal of developing a mutually agreed-upon formulation. (**For an example, see scenes 2–11 in the DVD.**)

Orientation

The therapist should orient the family members by letting them know what his or her purpose is for meeting with them and by finding out why each family member has come to the meeting, what each expects will happen during the session, and what they hope the outcome will be.

The therapist may start off by saying something such as: "I like to meet with the families of patients in order to find out how everybody sees what the problems are. This meeting will also give you an opportunity to ask questions. We will have a chance to discuss where to go from here and what next steps may be helpful."

An orientation normalizes the meeting as opposed to suggesting that there is something wrong with this particular family. The orientation empowers the family by letting them know that not only will they be asked questions but that they will also have the opportunity to ask questions. They are further empowered by the acknowledgment that they will be included in any decisions that may be made going forward.

The therapist continues with the following statements: "I would like to find out from each of you how you see what the problems are. I would like to know from each of you why you came today and what you hope to get out of this meeting." Once family members have expressed their opinions, the therapist condenses and feeds back their ideas to ensure that he or she has heard them and understood them as intended.

The therapist then expands on his or her goals for the meeting by letting the family know that he or she will be exploring further areas. For example, the therapist might say:

> "I would like to get a better idea about how you function as a family. This will give me a clearer understanding of your entire picture. Part of the reason that it is important to meet with all of you and understand how you function is that the way a family functions influences what happens to each family member. I am going to jump around a bit at times to find out about your family and ask a number of questions in different areas. Some questions may seem unrelated to the problems you are concerned about but they may be important. As we go along I will try to let you know what I am hearing to make sure that I have a correct impression of how you operate as a family. Does that make sense to you? Do you have any questions at this point?"

If the family has no questions and is in agreement, then the next step is to gather the necessary data. (**See scene 2 in the DVD.**)

Data Gathering

During this step, data are gathered about the presenting problems, overall family functioning, additional investigations, and other potential problems. The therapist asks family members what they think are the problems in the family. Each family member is asked his or her opinion. During this process the family learns to focus on specific issues, finds an outlet to express feelings, and establishes an atmosphere for listening and discussing. There are a number of challenges to gathering data efficiently. A balance has to be struck so as to obtain sufficient information to be able to arrive at a comprehensive and accurate formulation of the problem without getting bogged down in excessive details.

The therapist needs to gather enough information to clearly understand the problem, reformulate the problem to family members to make sure it is properly understood, but then limit further details about the problem to be able to move on to other problems. Another challenge to the data-gathering process is helping families learn to communicate and listen at the same time. In dysfunctional families there is a tendency for family members to interrupt each other to correct what the others are saying, to defend themselves, or to attack members who may appear to be critical of them. It is important that the therapist maintain control during this stage of the process in such a way as to validate each family member's perspective while at the same time helping the family to listen to each other without interruptions until everyone has had an opportunity to present his or her view. **(See scene 4 in the DVD.)**

Presenting problems.   The therapist begins by asking the family to describe the problem(s) that brought them to treatment. The therapist explores factual details, affective components of the problem, historical evolution of the problem, precipitating events, and who is involved in the problem and how. When the therapist feels that he or she has a good understanding of what family members are describing, it is helpful to summarize issues and check with the family as to whether they have in fact been correctly heard and understood. **(See scene 3 in the DVD.)**

Overall family functioning.   Once the presenting problem has been sufficiently and clearly delineated, the family's overall functioning needs to be assessed. The therapist can change the focus with the following statement: "Now I would like to get a general idea of how you operate as a family. Is that all right?"

At this point the therapist assesses the family along the six dimensions of the McMaster Model of Family Functioning: problem solving, communication, role allocation, affective responsiveness, affective involvement, and behavior control. The details of these dimensions and suggested questions for evaluating them are described in Chapter 4.

In brief, problem solving refers to a family's ability to resolve problems to a level that maintains effective family functioning. Communication refers to the verbal exchange of information within a family. Role allocation is the repetitive pattern of behavior by which family members fulfill family functions. Affective responsiveness evaluates the extent to which family members are able to respond with a full spectrum of feelings experienced in emotional life and whether the emotional experience is consistent or appropriate with the stimulant or situational context. Affective involvement is the extent to which the family shows interest in and values particular activities of individual family members. Behavior control refers to the pattern that families adopt for handling behaviors that may include situations that are physically dangerous, situations involving meeting and expressing psychobiological needs and drives, and situations involving socializing behaviors, both between family members and people outside the family system.

The assessment focuses on detailing strengths and difficulties in each of these areas of family life to determine aspects of overall family functioning that influence the emotional and/or physical health of family members. As each dimension is examined, the therapist should feed back to family members his or her understanding of both the assets and shortcomings evident in each particular area. The emphasis should be on strengths because these will be central to the therapeutic planning that will follow.

Dysfunctional transactional patterns.   Throughout the assessment stage the therapist needs to be aware of and recognize the occurrence of potentially dysfunctional transactional patterns. It is not necessary to deal with these transactional patterns early in the evaluation, particularly if it is likely to derail the assessment process. It is enough for the therapist to make note of the pattern and proceed with the rest of the assessment. Dysfunctional patterns tend to occur in association with the presenting problems and can be dealt with once the problem is more comprehensively understood. During the later stages of the assessment, if the therapist recognizes a consistent dysfunctional transactional pattern, then he or she may label the process directly and see if the family agrees with the observation. Alternatively, the therapist may question the family members regarding their observation of the transactional process and help them reflect about these interactions. (**See scene 5 in the DVD.**)

Additional investigation.   To arrive at a comprehensive biopsychosocial assessment, the therapist needs to gather information about biological systems, the intrapsychic status of individuals, value systems, and broader social systems such as school, work, and friendship networks. In the case of children, additional data that need to be gathered may include developmental history, pediatric examinations, psychological investigations, and school reports. For adults, the therapist may need to gather information concerning psychosocial history of the individual, a psychiatric examination, medical history, physical examination, and related laboratory and radiologic tests as appropriate. Psychological and neuropsychological assessments may also be important if relevant. Much of this information may need to be gathered outside of the assessment session itself. However, to arrive at a comprehensive biopsychosocial formulation, the therapist does need to obtain information about the biological, psychological, and social aspects of the presenting problem.

Before completing the assessment, the therapist needs to ask the family members if there are any additional problems or difficulties that have not yet been touched on. It is worth repeating that the time spent obtaining a comprehensive list of problems and sufficient data for the therapist to understand those problems is well spent, because incomplete evaluations are most likely to lead to resistance and to inadequate treatment.

Problem Description

By the time this stage is reached, the identified problems should be reasonably clear to the family and to the therapist, if the therapist has been diligent in checking out his or her assumptions with the family during the data gathering process. The purpose of the problem description step is to summarize the identified difficulties and to develop a formal list of problems to be addressed. The family and the therapist come to a mutual agreement about the problem list. The list can be made up of a series of unrelated problems or details of a particularly difficult problem. The therapist may add other problems to the list that he or she has identified during the assessment process either during the overall assessment of family functioning, observed transactional patterns that seem to be particularly disruptive, or information collected from additional investigations.

Problem Clarification

The final step in the assessment process is to obtain agreement regarding problems listed by the family and the therapist. Two types of disagreements may arise at this point. First, family members may disagree among themselves. In this case the therapist needs to attempt to negotiate a resolution of these differences or help the family to agree to disagree about the problems. If differences of opinion about the problem are relatively minor, the therapeutic process can proceed and the differences will likely resolve during the course of therapy. If differences of opinion are significant, then those differences need to be resolved before therapy can proceed. In such a case, the focus on resolving differences may be the first critical step in the therapy process.

The second type of disagreement may occur between the family and the therapist. Again, if the therapist considers that the difference is relatively minor in relation to the therapeutic issues, then the therapy may proceed or there may be agreement to disagree about the problems for the moment with the understanding that such differences will be monitored over time. If the therapy goes well, these disagreements usually dissolve in the course of dealing with more important issues.

In case of more fundamental disagreements between the therapist and the family, specific areas may need to be explored or the family may be asked to think about the differences for a period of time (1–2 weeks) and then return for more discussion. If the disagreement persists, the family might be offered a consultation with another therapist rather than termination. If the disagreement persists despite these attempts to come to a resolution, it is unlikely that the therapy between that particular therapist and that particular family will be successful.

Contracting

Substages of contracting

- Orientation
- Outlining options
- Negotiating expectations
- Contract signing

The second macro stage is contracting. The goal of this stage is to prepare a contract that delineates the expectations, goals, and commitments regarding therapy between family members and the therapist. The steps in this stage include orientation, outlining options, negotiating expectations, and contract signing.

Orientation

As with each stage, the first step in the process is to orient the family to this next phase of the treatment process to obtain their agreement to proceed. The therapist may say something such as: "If we agree on the problems, let's now discuss what can be done about them. Is that all right?"

Outlining Options

Each set of problems has a different set of options regarding possible ways of dealing with them. Nonetheless, there are generally four broad options from which family members can choose in dealing with any problem. First, the family can continue to function as before without attempting to bring about any change. Second, the family can attempt to work out their problems on their own without the help of a therapist. Third, the family can choose another type of treatment. Fourth, the family can agree to engage with the therapist in the current treatment format.

For each option, the therapist and family can discuss the pros and cons of taking that particular option. The therapist can be quite neutral in supporting a family's decision with regard to the choices made, except when the issue of safety is involved. Clearly, if somebody is significantly depressed and suicidal or if some type of physical or emotional abuse is likely to result from a poorly chosen option, the therapist needs to assert professional responsibility in ensuring that the appropriate treatment is recommended and, if it is rejected, that safeguards are put into place to ensure the safety of all family members.

Short of such dangerous situations, the therapist can help family members come to consensus about how they want to proceed with the agreed-upon problems determined during the assessment. The likelihood of a successful outcome for therapy will be greatly enhanced if family members proactively and of their own free will agree to engage in the treatment process. The corollary also holds true; if there is disagreement between the therapist and family members or between the family members themselves about the likelihood of commitment to the treatment process, it is unlikely that treatment will be successful. The therapist should not try to persuade or entice the family into treatment. If family members perceive that treatment is more important for the therapist than for the family, the likelihood of them engaging actively and collaboratively in the treatment process will be low. The therapist can make clear that he or she is in support of the family's choices even if it means not proceeding with family therapy. The therapist can also convey that if the family members change their mind in the future, the therapist will be available to help them at a later point when they feel more ready to commit to the change process. If the family chooses to continue with the treatment process, then the therapist can proceed to the next step.

Negotiating Expectations

The goal of the negotiating stage is to formulate a set of expectations that each family member wants to see occur if treatment is to be successful. These expectations should be stated in concrete, behavioral terms to allow for clearly identifying and assessing change. Goals such as "I want you to be happy" or "I want us all to get along" should be reformulated in a way that family members can change their behaviors leading to such goals. The behaviors should be observable to all family members. For instance, in the above example, the goals can be reformulated to such behavior as spending more time together, being more affectionate with each other, giving each other more positive feedback, and engaging in more pleasurable activities together, all behaviors that if carried out are likely to lead to the broader affective goals. The therapist and family should take each of the problems outlined in the assessment and develop a set of behavioral goals relating to those problems that, if carried out, will give the family a sense that they are making changes.

It may seem overwhelming to both therapist and family to set a large number of goals for problems, each with a number of subcomponents, as a way of trying to resolve them. In reality, as families change their pattern of dealing with each other around some of their problems, these newfound interactional processes generalize to many of the presenting problems, so that by the end of the process it may not be necessary to methodically work through each one.

The therapist also expresses his or her expectations of the family. These expectations usually revolve around the family's following through in keeping their appointments and attempting to make the changes they have agreed to. The therapist should also expect that there be no acting-out behavior, physical or sexual abuse, or suicidal threats during the course of treatment.

The main technique for establishing treatment goals is that family members negotiate what they would like from each other and how they want each other to change, in order to feel they have been successful in treatment. The family then is given the major responsibility for defining their expectations of each other. The therapist's primary role during this process is to facilitate the interaction between family members to ensure that clear, behaviorally defined expectations of change are established. The therapist should also make sure that expectations are realistic for the time frame the family has designated to make the changes. The therapist may also need to raise additional problems that are not addressed by the family during the negotiating process, particularly if the therapist feels those problems may be central to the ongoing difficulties that the family is experiencing. (**See scene 14 in the DVD.**)

Contract Signing

After the completion of the list of expectations from each family member and between the therapist and family, the therapist may prepare a written contract, which lists the problems and specifies what has been agreed on between participants. The therapist and family members then sign the contract. Generally, the family and therapist should aim to work on two or three tasks per session so as to not overload the family and to make success most likely.

The importance of a written contract can be debated. In general, it is helpful to have a written document of the expectations that family members have of each other. A written document emphasizes the importance of the treatment process. It also serves as a reminder to family members of what they have agreed on. Just as importantly, having the goals and expectations in written form eliminates the possibility of participants misinterpreting or misrepresenting what they thought had been said and agreed on in previous sessions. If there are not too many problems and if the goals that have been agreed on are relatively straightforward and clear, a written contract may be less important.

Treatment

Substages of treatment

- Orientation
- Clarifying priorities
- Setting tasks
- Task evaluation

The third macro stage is the treatment stage. The goals of the treatment stage are to develop and implement problem-solving strategies to change the identified problems. Two therapeutic techniques are used to accomplish these goals. The first is focused on producing behavioral change in the family through task setting. The therapist helps the family to set tasks that they can work on between meetings. Evaluation of the success or failure of the family in accomplishing these tasks becomes the main focus of the work in subsequent family sessions. The second set of techniques promotes cognitive and behavioral changes that are likely to increase the family's ability to address their problems successfully. The treatment stage consists of four steps: orientation, clarifying priorities, setting tasks, and task evaluation.

Orientation

The first step as usual is to orient the family to a new stage and to obtain their permission to proceed. The therapist can then say something like, "Now that we have agreed to work together, how would you like to begin?"

Clarifying Priorities

This step involves ordering the problem list to establish priorities. It is preferable to allow the family to establish the priority of problems to be dealt with to empower them and emphasize their responsibility for making decisions about how they want to function. If the family cannot establish priorities or has ignored urgent problems that the therapist feels need to be addressed, then the therapist should intervene to change the priority list. Examples of urgent problems that demand immediate action are suicidality, substance abuse, significant eating disorders, and physical or sexual abuse in the home.

In general, priority should be given to problems that involve communications and behavior control, because problems in these areas can lead to difficulties in solving other problems. If families cannot communicate about issues, it is going to be difficult for them to negotiate expectations. Similarly, if chaotic behavior is allowed to proceed, this is likely to disrupt treatment.

Setting Tasks

Task setting involves general and specific principles.

General principles.   Starting with the first problem prioritized by the family, the therapist asks the family to negotiate with each other what changes they would like from each other that, if carried out, would represent a move in the direction of meeting their expectations of change. Such behavioral changes are the tasks the family will be working on during the course of treatment. If family members are unable to come up with reasonable tasks and expectations from each other, the therapist may have to make some suggestions, checking with the family to ensure that they are agreeable to everyone.

In negotiating and assigning tasks, the therapist should consider the following general principles:

1. The therapist should be open and direct with the family about the purpose of the assigned tasks. Often it is not the specific task that is important but the fact that family members are making an effort to meet each other's needs in a way that is different from their usual patterns. The task should be direct and purposeful and not paradoxical. The idea is not to back the family into change but to have them move toward it in a proactive and purposeful manner.
2. Tasks should be directed toward bringing about change in those dimensions of family functioning that have been identified as problematic during the assessment process.
3. Tasks should be directed at changing dysfunctional family transactional patterns.
4. Following the principles of shaping, initial tasks should be simple and achievable to increase their potential for success. As the family gains confidence in themselves and are empowered by the process of change, more complicated tasks can be negotiated.
5. Tasks should be reasonable with regard to age, gender, and sociocultural norms for that family.
6. Tasks should be oriented toward increasing positive behaviors rather than decreasing negative ones.
7. Task should be behavioral and concrete enough to be understood and evaluated by family members.
8. Tasks should be meaningful and important to the family.
9. Family members should feel that they could accomplish the tasks assigned to them, making it likely that they will commit themselves to carrying them out.
10. Emotionally oriented tasks should emphasize positive, not negative, feelings.

11. Tasks should fit reasonably into the family's schedule of activities.
12. A limited number of tasks per session should be assigned so that the family is not overloaded. A maximum of two tasks per session is usually reasonable.
13. Assignment of tasks to family members should be balanced so that major responsibility for completing tasks does not reside with one or two members.
14. Vindictiveness and rehashing of the past should be avoided and focus should be placed on constructive ways of dealing with the current situation.

These principles are made explicit to the family when the tasks are being negotiated. For instance, if one spouse indicates that he or she wants the other to "stop being so negative," the therapist may reframe expectations with a statement such as "It's understandable that you would like that, but it is usually harder to ask someone to stop doing something than to start doing something. What could he do for or with you during this coming week that would make you feel more positively connected to him?"

Once tasks have been assigned, it is useful to designate a family member to monitor and report on the performance of the family at working on the tasks at the next therapy session. Designating a monitor can increase the sense of involvement by family members in their own treatment and further localizes control for the change process within the family in terms of responsibility and accountability. The role of the monitor may be rotated among members or may vary with tasks. (**For an example of task setting, see scene 14 in the DVD.**)

Specific principles.   There are specific types of tasks that may be useful in the various dimensions of family functioning as described in the McMaster Model.

Problem solving: If the family is found to have difficulty solving problems, the following tasks may be helpful in bringing about constructive change. If the family has trouble identifying problems, then a family member can be assigned the task of bringing information about potential problems to the following session for the family to review. If families can identify problems but have difficulty coming to some decision about how to resolve them, then family members can work out a way of assigning individual members the responsibility of developing a list of alternative solutions to a particular problem. Another task for a family may be to discuss the pros and cons of the problem-solving options outlined to see if they can come to a mutual satisfactory decision. Finally, family members can monitor actions directed toward the resolution of the problem to generate feedback about which aspects of the process worked or did not work.

Communication: If communication is a problem within the family, the most common task is to have the family negotiate spending a set amount of time together talking about particular issues. Initially, families should only attempt to do this for a short period of time (5–10 minutes) and mostly about practical and instrumental rather than emotionally charged issues. Topics can range from discussing what happened during the day to positive experiences in the past to aspirations for the future. A specific time should be designated in advance for when this discussion can best take place. When family members are able to discuss nonthreatening instrumental issues successfully, they may try to talk more gradually about feelings, initially positive feelings, before attempting to discuss feelings with much more charged affect.

Family members can also be helped to address each other directly, to listen to each other, to let each other know that they have been heard and what they heard, and to agree to disagree about some issues. The duration of the time that family members spend talking to each other can be gradually increased as they become more comfortable with the process.

Role allocation: In families that have difficulties in apportioning responsibilities in a way that feels fair to all members, one task may be to have the family negotiate responsibilities from a list of necessary family roles and functions. Families should be careful to make sure that the responsibilities assigned to individuals are appropriate to their age and other roles within the family. Families can also be encouraged to develop a way of determining accountability for members' following through on what they have agreed to take on as new roles or responsibilities. Families may also need to discuss how they would deal with members who do not fulfill their agreed-upon responsibilities.

Affective responsiveness: This dimension focuses on appropriate ways for family members to manage emergency and welfare emotions. Emergency emotions refer to rage, anger, and aggression; welfare emotions refer to warmth, empathy, and caring.

As a way of helping families develop greater connection through welfare affect, partners can agree to do simple things such as kiss and/or hug each other on leaving or returning home. Setting time aside for family members to say positive and supportive things to each other, to hold or stroke each other, compliment each other, and respond positively to such reaching out can be negotiated. Although this kind of activity may seem superficial and contrived at first, positive output by family members tends to stimulate similar responses from others over time.

Tasks for coping with emergency emotions such as rage, anger, and aggression center around helping individuals overcome their fear of feeling and expressing anger. Family members can practice recognizing and anticipating anger-provoking situations and escalating processes before such negative affect gets out of control. Individuals can then practice how to express their anger in a more calm and constructive manner. Family members can practice disengaging from situations that have in the past led to inevitable escalation of destructive affect.

Affective involvement: It is common for either lack of involvement or overinvolvement of family members with each other to be a problem in this dimension. For lack of involvement, family members can set aside specific times each week when members get together to talk or participate in joint activities that each family member finds pleasurable. For overinvolvement, tasks can be set up that allow for greater separation and autonomy by members to do things without the supervision or intrusion of other members. The family can learn to modulate the amount of time and level of intensity in their interactions with each other.

Behavior control: Overcontrol or undercontrol are the usual problems in this dimension. For undercontrol, tasks that increase the clarity of expectations between family members' responsibilities and ways of doing things can be set. The family can discuss these expectations and set contingencies in case they are not carried out. All members should be involved in the process of determining what are acceptable behaviors and acceptable contingencies in case of noncompliance. In overcontrolling situations, the task is to help families negotiate a lesser level of control and to practice allowing more autonomy for family members. In setting tasks for behavior control, the most important issues are to make sure family members adhere to their own expectations concerning rules and standards, spelling out rewards and sanctions clearly, and making sure that the agreed-upon processes are followed through.

Task Evaluation

Task evaluation is a critical process. This is the crux of the therapeutic work. It is in the review of the family's success or failure in carrying out their tasks that the real issues in the family become manifest. The tasks, apart from their intrinsic value, are a stimulus for core family issues to emerge and become more evident, not only to the therapist but also to the family members through the eyes of the therapist. Obstacles in carrying out agreed-upon tasks become stimuli and catalysts for bringing about subsequent changes. The ways in which families have difficulty accomplishing tasks provide the best immediate evidence of what the family needs to work on. Failure to accomplish tasks should not be seen by the therapist or the family as an obstacle to change but as an opportunity to gain a much clearer insight into the problems of the family in a more immediate, nonintellectual, and effective manner. If the family is committed to the change process, awareness of the particular ways in which they run into obstacles in carrying out their tasks allows them to make more constructive and effective changes.

If the agreed-upon tasks are accomplished, the therapist provides positive reinforcement, reviewing and highlighting the positive aspects of the family's performance to ensure that the family members understand what worked so they can continue to resolve problems in the future. If the tasks are not accomplished or only partially accomplished, the therapist needs to go through the particular steps in some detail to find out what went wrong. Failure to accomplish a task provides important information about difficulties that may not have been fully articulated during the assessment process.

In addition to reviewing the specifics of the family's attempt to accomplish a failed task, it is also important to determine whether the task was too difficult for that particular family. If the task was too difficult, a simpler task, broken down into smaller, more manageable pieces, may be needed. It is also possible that a task may have failed owing to difficulties that were not apparent during previous assessments. In this case, knowledge of the new difficulties can be incorporated in the formulation of the family's problems and in the setting of new tasks. A failed task may also indicate to the therapist that his or her formulation of the problem was incorrect and that the identified problem is associated with other factors not previously considered. In this case, again, the therapist needs to reformulate the problem in a way that allows for a more effective treatment plan.

Finally, a failed task may mean that the family is not interested in working to bring about change. They may have changed their minds about their commitment to therapy, or they may decide that the amount of effort involved is too great. If noncompliance is the key reason for the failure of tasks, this needs to be addressed with the family to determine if they are invested enough in the treatment process to make treatment succeed. In general, unless there is a dangerous situation involved, it is more important for the family to obtain good results in therapy than it should be for the therapist. If families are not willing to work as hard as they need to in order to bring about change, this should be reflected back to them. If they are not ready to commit to the treatment process, they should be offered the opportunity to return to the therapist at some future date if and when they decide they are ready for the effort they will need to put into the treatment. This information can be offered in a supportive way, indicating that success comes with true commitment when the family has the time and energy to enter treatment.

An example of the application of these principles is shown in scenes 17 and 18 of the accompanying DVD. The scenes show a comprehensive family evaluation, negotiation of expectations, task assignment, and task evaluation. The Appendix at the end of Chapter 4 contains a write-up of the family assessment and the task assignments chosen by the family. Appendix 9–1 at the end of this chapter outlines the format of the treatment.

Other Techniques

During the treatment stage, the major part of each session is devoted to reviewing previously assigned tasks and developing and negotiating new tasks. There are some specific intervention tools that can help the therapist and family negotiate their way through the process of bringing about meaningful change.

Clarification of problems: One ongoing way of engaging the family and encouraging change is for the therapist to clarify the family's problems in such a way that the problem as well as antecedents and consequences are understood and agreed on by family members. The therapist's feedback provides clear descriptions of his or her perception of the family's functioning. The assumption is that if families understand themselves better, they are more likely to make those changes. Clarification of problems helps families become aware of processes in the family patterns of organization that may not have been clear to them and may have created problems that can be changed. As in individual psychotherapy, the assumption is that with sufficient knowledge about oneself or one's system, change will more readily take place.

Labeling and interpreting of transactions: The therapist can also teach recognition skills as he or she labels and interprets dysfunctional transactional patterns during therapy sessions. As with the clarification of problems, it is assumed that if families understand their transactional patterns and can evaluate them more effectively, it brings these patterns more within their control, either to change them or to accept them without attributing undue meaning to them. The therapist can also label unacknowledged affect that may occur during these transactional patterns. Labeling and interpreting of process is based on observable behaviors that occur during the therapy sessions, therefore making them more immediate and real. By learning to understand the transactional patterns, families can either modify them to be less destructive or harness them in the service of bringing about more effective functioning.

Psychoeducation: Families in which one or more member has an identified psychiatric (medical) problem often have inaccurate assumptions, expectations, and information about the disorder, its consequences, and its treatment. Providing the family with information about the disorder, its etiology, course, and treatment may help eliminate misunderstanding and empower the family to develop better coping skills for managing the illness.

Closure

Substages of closure

- Orientation
- Summary of treatment
- Long-term goals
- Follow-up

The final macro stage is closure and consists of four steps: orientation, summary of treatment, long-term goals, and follow-up.

Orientation

During the orientation step, the therapist points out to the family that expectations as set forth in the contract have been met and that the therapy can now end. If the family wants to continue with further therapy, this needs to be explored and renegotiated. If the family members have met their goals, they should be encouraged to try to resolve new issues that come up using their new coping skills and call for help if they run into significant problems they cannot resolve on their own. It is important not to make professional patients out of families by keeping them too dependent on the therapist.

Summary of Treatment

Family members should be asked to summarize what has happened during treatment and what they have learned. The therapist then confirms or elaborates on their perceptions and adds any insights that may have been overlooked. The therapist should also check at this point what the family intends to do should any of their problems recur. In this step, problems and solutions are reviewed and steps for remediation should relapse occur are discussed and put into place.

Long-Term Goals

The therapist at this point asks the family to discuss and set long-term goals. Family members are asked to identify issues they anticipate might come up or prove problematic in the future. The family is supported in recognizing that they have been able to make significant gains and that they have developed effective ways of identifying and dealing with family problems. Having said this, the therapist reassures the family that they have the option of returning for additional help when and if it is needed.

Follow-Up

Therapy ends at this point, although for some families an intermittent follow-up schedule may be appropriate. This could be at 3, 6, or 9 months. When a follow-up visit is arranged, it should be set far enough in the future to allow the family a full opportunity to deal with issues as they arise. The follow-up session should also support and monitor progress rather than rehash issues that have already been dealt with effectively.

Conclusion

In most cases, the effectiveness of the therapeutic process reflects a degree of thoroughness and rigor that the therapist maintains by systematically following the major treatment stages and the subcomponent steps. This includes adhering to the principle of keeping the family actively involved in working with the therapist at each step of the treatment process. The therapist learns to function as an assessor, evaluator, diagnostician, clarifier, investigator, catalyst, facilitator, and at times confronter. The therapist must be prepared to give major responsibility for treatment to the family while remaining intently involved in the treatment process. The therapist needs be able to delegate increased responsibility to the family as family members learn to work on their own problems. The therapist needs to be able to terminate therapy when there is sufficient evidence that the family is not attempting to resolve their problems. The therapist, needless to say, must demonstrate ongoing commitment to the change process by remaining integrally involved in monitoring and providing feedback about his or her observations regarding the family's attempts to deal with their problems throughout the full course of treatment.

References

1. Epstein NB, Bishop DS: Problem-Centered Systems Therapy of the Family. J Marital Fam Ther 7: 23–31, 1981
2. Epstein NB, Bishop DS, Levin S: The McMaster model of family functioning. J Marriage Fam Couns 4:19–31, 1978
3. Tomm KM, Wright LM: Training in family therapy: perceptual, conceptual, and executive skills. Fam Process 18:227–250, 1979

Appendix 9–1. Case Example

The Treatment Stage

Please refer to the DVD. See the Appendix to Chapter 4 for a description of the assessment of this family.

At the completion of the assessment process, the family negotiates expectations from each other in terms of tasks that they agree to undertake. These tasks address some of the concerns that the family has identified as being problematic for them. Working on these tasks signifies the willingness of family members to make changes to improve their relationships.

As indices of their commitment to improve ways of connecting and interacting with each other, the family agrees to the following first steps (see also Chapter 4):

Wife's requests:
- The husband to be at the dinner table at the agreed-upon time.
- The husband and wife to spend one half day of each weekend doing something together.

Husband's requests:
- Over dinner, the wife to talk about their day as opposed to focusing on problems with their children or her depressed mood.
- The wife to greet him when he comes home and ask about how his day went.

Parents' requests of daughter:
- Clean her room or close the door.
- Do her own laundry.

Daughter's request of parents:
- Take care of each other's needs better so that she does not feel the need to provide for them what they are not getting from each other.

Tasks Successfully Accomplished

The family was partially successful in accomplishing some of their goals. The father was mostly on time for meals. The mother often asked about the father's day and was positive during supper. The daughter kept her door closed and attempted to do her own laundry. The therapist acknowledged these successes and praised the family for their efforts.

Tasks Not Accomplished

The daughter left her clothes in the washing machine after using it. The father was not always on time for dinner. The mother did not always greet him when he came home from work. The husband and wife had an argument about how to spend their weekend time together.

The therapist has to determine the reason for their failure. Was it because they misunderstood the particulars of their agreement? Do family members feel ambivalent or mistrustful of making changes? The therapist helps the family to understand the reasons for not being successful and helps them to clarify expectations as they work toward fulfilling their commitments to each other.

This process of task setting, task evaluation, and renegotiation is the working-through phase of the treatment. Families become more aware of both their strengths and their limitations by working on specific problems. The goal is for the family to learn to be able to problem solve on their own.

10

Integrating Family Treatment Into Biopsychosocial Care

- Optimal treatment should be based on a comprehensive understanding of the patient attained by completing a biopsychosocial (BPS) assessment.
- A BPS assessment consists of an assessment of biological, psychological, and social factors and includes attention to the culture, spirituality, and family context of the patient and the presenting problems.
- Psychiatrists are in a unique position to develop a BPS formulation and provide BPS treatment.

Care based on a truly integrated biopsychosocial (BPS) assessment has not been well studied. Most studies on integrated care refer to "combined" treatment, meaning the combination of psychotherapy and psychopharmacology, rather than comprehensive BPS treatment. However, in the provision of care, pragmatics is often the deciding principle, depending on factors such as the patient's financial resources and what treatment providers are available. This chapter reviews the evidence for BPS treatment in general and then specifically addresses the integration of family treatment into BPS care.

Evidence-Based Studies of Combined Treatment

Gabbard and Kay (1) describe combined treatment as the essence of psychiatric practice and the most obvious example of the BPS foundation on which treatment decisions are based. The studies they reviewed describe combined treatment as treatment in which two providers, in parallel, provide two separate and distinct treatments. In these studies, the treatment providers are highly trained psychotherapists and pharmacotherapists who utilize manuals and make treatment decisions for that specific modality only. This treatment is also referred to as split treatment or co-treatment. Rarely do any studies assess family treatment; combined treatment is generally understood as combining individual psychotherapy and psychopharmacology.

Combined treatment for major depression is associated with only a small improvement in efficacy (2). Nevertheless, other studies report positive outcomes with faster results (3), lower relapse rates (4, 5, 6), better long-term social adjustment (7), and lower relapse rates after discontinuation of treatment (8). Trends suggest that adding psychotherapy to antidepressant medication may be particularly effective for patients with severe or chronic depression. Otto and colleagues (9) state that combined treatment for major depression may have beneficial effects when applied to patients with chronic depression and to prevent relapse. However, for mild to moderate major depressive disorder, a good response occurs with either medication or psychotherapy (10, 11). Despite much enthusiasm for the combined treatment of major depression, there are consistent differences in outcome, resulting in a range of conclusions regarding the efficacy of combined treatment.

For other illnesses, treatment that includes a variety of modalities has variable results. For bipolar disorder, treatment that includes family treatment improves long-term outcome (12). For schizophrenia, patients living alone have a higher relapse rate when psychotherapy is added (13). For anxiety disorder, there are some benefits in the short term for combined treatment, but combined treatment may limit the maintenance of treatment gains offered by cognitive-behavioral therapy (CBT) alone (9). For panic disorder, adding an antidepressant to CBT is better than either modality alone, although a benzodiazepine does not improve outcome (14).

Overall, combined treatment is more effective than single-modality treatment, the effect sizes are generally modest, and differences that are statistically significant may not be clinically meaningful. Given the added strain of providing combined treatment on limited mental health resources, can therapists selectively provide combined treatment to those patients most likely to show a significant benefit?

Combined and integrated treatment

- **Combined treatment:** two therapists, in parallel, provide two distinct treatments
- **Integrated treatment:** one therapist provides the various treatments

In summary, certain patients show a better response to combined treatment than single-modality treatment. These are patients with more severe depression (3, 15, 16), endogenous depression (17), chronic depression (8, 18), and dysfunctional cognitions (15). If patients have a poor response to single-modality treatment, they may do better with combined treatment (19, 20).

Why Is Combined Treatment Better in Some Cases?

Some benefit may accrue simply from additive effects. Each treatment that is effective in its own right can show a cumulative effect when combined. Functional neuroimaging of the differential effects of psychotherapy and antidepressant medications suggests that, while both treatments show considerable overlap in effects on cerebral metabolism, medication effects develop "bottom up," emanating from the brain stem upward, whereas psychotherapy effects emerge in a "top-down" fashion, spreading downward from the frontal cortex (21). The two modalities may then exert an additive effect by addressing different symptom domains. Therapy, for example, might address the hopelessness related to depression, whereas medications may more directly address neurovegetative aspects of depression (22).

Interactive effects can also contribute to the increased efficacy of combined treatment. Pharmacotherapy can make some patients more available for therapy by easing treatment-interfering problems such as psychosis, disabling anxiety, or the motivational syndrome of depression. Psychotherapy enhances the effectiveness of medication by supporting compliance (23, 24, 25, 26) and enhancing patient satisfaction with treatment (25, 27). In a multicenter study funded by the National Institute of Mental Health for the treatment of depression, the strength of the patient-physician alliance was associated with the best treatment outcome, even when patients received placebo (28).

Benefits of combined treatment

- More effective for severe forms of illness
- Helpful when single-modality treatment has not been sufficiently effective
- Maximizes additive and interactive ingredients of different treatments

---

What About Offering Treatments Sequentially?

Administration of treatments in a sequential order is a common practice in clinical medicine but is rarely done in psychiatry. Fava et al. (29) conducted a review of clinical trials in which treatment components were used in a sequential order with mixed results. In recurrent depression, the sequential use of pharmacotherapy was found to reduce relapse rate. In bipolar disorder, the use of psychotherapeutic strategies in patients who were already undergoing treatment with mood stabilizers yielded clinical benefits. In anxiety disorders, the sequential use of pharmacotherapy and psychotherapy was not found to improve long-term outcome.

What Are the Best Ways to Combine Treatments?

The literature also refers to integration of care and integrated treatment, two models that combine care in different ways. Integration of care occurs at an organizational level when patients receive co-coordinated treatment with several components delivered by several providers that are coordinated by an overseer of care. Integration of care frequently includes a family component, usually family psychoeducation. Integrated treatment describes a specific type of treatment in which the various treatment modalities are delivered by one provider. Both integration of care and integrated treatment are shown to have benefit for patients with multiple diagnoses.

Integration of Care

Integration of care for dual-diagnosis patients is strongly recommended (30) and is recognized by the Substance Abuse and Mental Health Services Administration as a consensus best practice (31). Integration of care for dually diagnosed patients produces fewer hospitalizations and lower arrest rates compared with parallel treatments (32). In Mangrum and colleagues' study (32), patients accessed substance abuse treatment, psychiatric services, individual therapy, and specialized groups tailored to dually diagnosed patients. Assertive engagement is practiced, involving the patient in treatment wherever this is most applicable. Patients in the parallel treatment condition received traditional independent substance abuse and mental health treatment through separate clinics without a centralized case management component overseeing care. Where a family component was offered, an additional benefit occurred with a decrease in the severity of psychiatric symptoms.

Integration of care for patients with depression improves outcome (33). Essential components of this program include engaging the patient in self-management, assessing for suicide, providing educational tools, and discussing barriers to care. Integration of care can be provided in an inpatient setting (34) with three phases of depression management: remoralization, remediation (or symptoms reduction), and rehabilitation and relapse prevention. In the remoralization phase, patient and family education occurs and hopes for recovery are actively promoted. In the remediation phase, patient mindfulness and patient and family friendliness are key, with specific techniques of stress reduction and behavioral techniques used along with medications. During the rehabilitation and relapse prevention phase, patients are expected to be active, and realistic expectations are discussed with the patient and the family to cope with remaining depressive symptoms and to reduce the risk of relapse. This model is illustrative of a true BPS treatment, although no current evidence exists regarding its efficacy.

Integration of care for patients with bipolar disorder improves outcome compared with treatment as usual (35). Significant treatment components include enhancing patient self-management skills with psychoeducation, providing clinicians with simplified practice guidelines, and improving patient access to care. Care coordinators ensure continuity of care and good information flow. The patients in the collaborative care program had fewer weeks of illness, reduced length of illness episode, improvement in social role function, better quality of life, and greater treatment satisfaction. The intervention was cost-neutral. Most benefits accrued in the 2nd and 3rd years.

The commonalities to the systems of integration of care include one overseer, active engagement of the patient, psychoeducation, and intelligent application of treatment according to the patient's current needs. Within integration-of-care models, care may be provided by several providers, but the approach is closely coordinated by the program director. Minkoff and Cline (31) state, "Empathic, hopeful, integrated treatment relationships are one of the most important contributors to treatment success in any setting" (p. 731).

Integrated Treatment

Integrated treatment is the provision of the necessary components of treatment, whether biological, psychological, and/or social, by one provider. In contrast, combined care is usually delivered by more than one provider. Coordination of care by regular communication between different therapists is necessary for optimal combined care but often does not take place routinely in real-world clinical practice because of time constraints and reimbursement limitations. Integrated treatment eliminates the potential problems of therapists working at cross-purposes or of the patient overvaluing one therapist while undervaluing the other (splitting). A single therapist is able to more readily acquire a comprehensive knowledge of the patient, knowledge that can better inform a treatment plan and put into perspective difficulties that may arise during the course of treatment.

Psychiatrist-delivered integrated treatment describes a specific type of treatment that includes all necessary elements of care delivered exclusively by a psychiatrist. In contrast, combined or split treatment is care divided between two providers, usually a psychopharmacologist and a psychotherapist. Psychiatrist-delivered integrated treatment for patients with depression resulted in fewer outpatient sessions and lower treatment costs compared with patients receiving treatment delivered by two providers (36).

Gabbard and Kay (1) recognize the benefits of one-person delivered care: "Like surgeons, who are trained to know when they should not operate, psychiatrists are trained to know when they should not prescribe, and their knowledge allows them to think about patients from the dual perspective of both biology and psychology in all clinical encounters" (p. 1957). The authors also point out the demands of a one-person treatment model: "the psychiatrist must think both in terms of a dysfunctional brain and a psychologically distressed human being. The psychiatrist must be capable of shifting from a more or less objective and observational perspective to an empathic, intersubjective (but no less scientific) approach. While this balancing act is challenging, it is also the essence of good medical and psychiatric practice, epitomizing Engel's biopsychosocial model. The psychiatrist, like any other good physician, treats the whole person" (p. 1959). The authors note that "biological reductionism may appeal to all of us when immersing ourselves in human suffering is too much to bear. An exclusive focus on dosage adjustment and side effects may provide the psychiatrist with a buffer against painful empathic awareness of the patient's despair as well as offering an illusion of mastery over the complexities of psychiatric illness" (p. 1959). (**The DVD describes the biopsychosocial approach in scene 15.**)

Benefits and shortcomings of integrated treatment

Benefits
- Better understanding of the illness and its context
- More consistent care
- Better coordination of care
- More cost-effective

Shortcomings
- Need for broad skills base
- More time-consuming
- Neutrality more difficult to maintain
- Greater potential for breaching confidentiality

How Does the Psychiatrist Deliver Integrated Treatment?

Glick (37) offers guidelines to psychiatrists for the integration of pharmacotherapy with psychotherapeutic management, calling it *multimodal therapy*. He describes this treatment as follows: After diagnosis has been reached, goals as targets for improvement are selected. These goals then determine which treatment modality is used. The sequence of therapies can vary according to clinical considerations regarding the type of illness, its severity, and the clinician-patient concept of the nature of the illness. In psychosis, the physician medicates first, then adds family therapy and/or individual psychotherapy. If one modality is effective, there is no need for a second modality. For some situations, starting with family therapy makes the most clinical sense; for others, with individual therapy. In other situations, one may want to start several treatments simultaneously. One modality can be withdrawn as the problems that initiated that treatment resolve. One treatment may resolve the illness, but comorbidity such as alcoholism may necessitate a second treatment. In addition, family psychoeducation can increase medication compliance. This approach requires the psychiatrist to have a broad skill base and experience to know what is needed. There have been studies that compare multimodal therapy with treatment delivered by several providers.

Psychiatrist-delivered integrated treatment

- The psychiatrist has to be comfortable with multiple roles
- The psychiatrist must be acceptable to the patient and family
- The psychiatrist needs to pay special attention to boundaries and confidentiality

---

Single-provider integrated treatment is cheaper than multiple-provider or split treatment (36, 38). Treatments in which the pharmacologic work is seen to support the therapy and the therapy supports the drug treatment may be the most integrated, as with the model of psychodynamic psychopharmacology developed by Mintz et al. (39) in which the therapist understands problems with medication (e.g., noncompliance, fear of dependency, a tendency to develop side effects) as targets for psychotherapeutic exploration.

Many psychiatrists will not be interested in, be trained sufficiently, or find it financially feasible to provide integrated treatment. These psychiatrists, however, should still meet with the families of their patients. At a minimum such meetings will provide valuable information needed for a BPS understanding of the patient and the presenting problems. Meeting with a family will also likely improve collaboration, compliance, and support for the treatment process. There is clear evidence that involving the family improves patient outcome for many illnesses (see Chapters 3 and 11). However, little has been written about how the psychiatrist can do this, especially concerning clinical decision making. Questions of confidentiality, boundaries, how to combine treatment, and when to combine treatment often appear overwhelming to a psychiatrist with little training in this area. Next, we describe when and how to involve the family in patient care.

When Does the Clinician Involve the Family?

It is reasonable to try to determine when it is cost-effective to involve the family in the treatment of a patient with a psychiatric disorder. Involving the family in treatment makes the most sense when there is evidence to support the additional benefit of family interventions in the course and outcome of a particular disorder. Although there are studies that show the effectiveness of an adjunctive family therapy in the management of a variety of psychiatric disorders, including mood disorders, schizophrenia, anxiety disorders, and organic brain syndromes, the amount of additional benefit to be derived is not always obvious.

There are many ways in which illnesses can be treated. There are also many types of outcomes that can be evaluated and deemed relevant. Outcome can be defined as improvement in symptoms, improvement in work functioning, improvement in social functioning, improvement in quality of life, improvement in life satisfaction and meaning of life, or cost-effectiveness. The usefulness of family interventions may depend on which of the outcomes outlined above are seen as being most important or relevant.

The available evidence for the effectiveness of a variety of treatments is limited. It is therefore important to be as comprehensive as possible in the assessment and treatment of patients, to be efficient, and above all to do no harm. The BPS perspective describes a systematic evaluation of the relevant variables likely to be influencing the onset and course of a disorder without overemphasizing any single aspect of the disorder. Harm may be caused by a too-narrow formulation of the problem, whether biological (leading to polypharmacy), psychological (too much emphasis on distorted cognitions or dynamic conflicts), or social (blaming the family). For most serious psychiatric disorders, it makes good clinical sense to formulate the problem in a way that allows for an evaluation of the biological, psychological, and social dimensions, which in turn informs a BPS treatment plan.

When the BPS formulation is generated, the clinician can then determine what the relative contributions of these components are for that particular patient. The case of the chronically depressed suicidal patient with borderline personality disorder described in Chapter 5 provides a good example. From a biological perspective, this patient has a genetic vulnerability to depression due to a significant family history of mood disorders and to the chronic nature of her depression. From a psychological perspective, the patient is struggling with the sequelae of childhood sexual abuse, including low self-esteem, self-hatred and blame, conflict over dependence and independence, and its effect on her sexual functioning. From a social perspective, she has significant family dysfunction secondary to poor communication and problem-solving skills, a lack of well-defined expectations about acceptable standards of behavior in the family, and uncertainty about emotional connectedness. By formulating the patient's presentation from this broad perspective, the psychiatrist can shape her treatment to include pharmacotherapy, individual psychotherapy, and family intervention without unduly relying on any one of those treatment modalities.

Addressing the major influences on the onset and course of the disorder, the psychiatrist is most likely to find the combination of treatments that meets the greatest needs. A broad formulation also makes good common sense to the patient and his or her family. They feel reassured, understood, and empowered to make changes in what was previously seen as an overwhelming situation. Bringing clarity into a seemingly emotionally charged and confusing situation can be very therapeutic in and of itself. Such clarity is most likely to be achieved when all the relevant factors affecting the presenting problem(s) are identified. **Part One of the DVD when viewed in its entirety illustrates how to assess a family of a patient with chronic depressive symptoms. The Commentary on Assessment (scene 15) and the Commentary on Treatment (scene 19) illustrate the philosophical underpinnings of the McMaster Model and the Problem-Centered Systems Therapy of the Family (PCSTF).** The use of a broad BPS formulation helps the family make sense of a confusing and overwhelming situation. This clarity then allows the family to feel empowered to make changes.

However, not all presenting problems need a multimodal treatment plan. A comprehensive evaluation may determine that there is no need for multiple treatments and in fact may uncover specific strengths that can be mobilized within the family. Not all patients need pharmacotherapy, individual psycho-therapy, or family therapy. The combination of useful treatments should be determined by their relevance to the presenting problem.

Which Treatment to Choose?

Once a range of treatments is decided on, there are many options. Biological treatments include pharmacotherapy, electroconvulsive therapy, and vagus nerve stimulation. Psychological treatments include cognitive-behavioral therapy, interpersonal therapy, dynamic therapy, or supportive psychotherapy. Family therapies include structural therapy, strategic therapy, and the problem-centered systems therapy, among others. Choosing any one of these options based on available evidence is difficult. In general, there is no good evidence to prove that any form of therapy is consistently better than another, although certain treatments have been shown to be somewhat more effective than others for certain disorders in certain populations. There are, however, too many unknown mediating variables, including therapist competence, patient preference, timing of the intervention, responsiveness of a particular illness, comorbidity, and the current social situation, to be able to make definitive recommendations that transcend these variables.

Regarding family therapies, given the current lack of evidence about efficacy, the therapist should choose the particular type of family therapy he or she is most comfortable with and best trained in and that fits his or her theoretical preference and personality style. Although it is useful to have a reasonably wide range of possible approaches available to the therapist, there is a risk of borrowing from different treatment models without learning how to do any one of them systematically and consistently, as well as mixing interventions that may conflict with each other. In this book we advocate two practices as part of routine patient care: to complete a BPS assessment and treatment plan and to use the PCSTF treatment approach when such an approach is needed.

Who Should Provide the Different Therapies?

Opinions vary regarding not only the feasibility and advisability of combining pharmacological, psychological, and family treatments but also the ways these treatments may be best delivered. Should treatments be provided by one provider? Two providers? Three providers? What are the advantages and disadvantages of having fewer or more therapists?

In reality, only a psychiatrist can provide all three modalities—pharmacotherapy, psychotherapy, and family therapy—to a patient. The current trend is for different treatments to be provided by different therapists. It is quite common for a psychiatrist to provide medication management, an individual therapist to provide psychotherapy, and a family therapist to work with the family. Some disciplines explicitly discourage therapists from treating both an individual and his or her family. This separation of boundaries clearly reduces potential conflicts of interest and distrust by patients and families about disclosure of confidential information. Therapists may also become more proficient in their therapeutic skills if they restrict treatment to only one modality. It is difficult to be an expert in multiple forms of treatment. Providing too many forms of treatment to the same individual and family may also be too time-consuming for any one provider, decreasing the provider's availability to other patients.

However, there are good reasons why the same provider should provide different treatments to the same patient and his or her family. One reason is for ease and coordination of treatment. In addition, it is difficult to discuss ongoing treatment issues with different therapists on a regular basis, given limited time for such discussions and the fact that coordination time is not reimbursable. The potential for splitting is also eliminated when there is only one provider. Further, there is less likelihood of patients and families being confused by different conceptual frameworks when one provider provides integrated care. In addition to consistency of style, a single provider using multiple treatment modalities is more likely to have a broader overview and more thorough understanding of the issues influencing the presenting problem.

Case Examples

These cases illustrate how different combinations of treatments by different therapists may be suitable at different times depending on patients' needs, therapists' availability, and specific components of the presenting problems.

Deborah W

Deborah W first presented for psychiatric treatment to an inpatient unit during a manic episode at age 19. She had a history of bipolar disorder beginning at age 16. A family meeting was held during her hospitalization to better understand the onset and course of her illness and to evaluate whether family issues may have played a role in the current presentation. Subsequent to her hospitalization, Deborah returned to the university while continuing to live at home. She was followed as an outpatient by a psychiatrist who in addition to pharmacotherapy worked with her in psychotherapy on the meaning of her illness and its impact on her sense of self and on her relationships with others. Deborah's family had difficulty understanding and coping with her illness, and the psychiatrist held a number of meetings with the family, including her parents and two siblings. These meetings focused on educating family members about bipolar disorder and helping them to work out more effective ways of dealing with it. During these meetings, it became evident that Deborah's parents had significant marital problems relating to her father's worsening drinking. Her parents asked to see the psychiatrist for couples therapy. Couples therapy resulted in a mutual decision by the parents to separate. Both parents then requested individual sessions to help them to cope with the separation process. The psychiatrist also continued to meet with Deborah during this time to manage her illness and help her deal with her parents' divorce.

Deborah eventually completed a college degree and started working; her parents both remarried. She continued to have multiple episodes of mood disorder requiring changes in pharmacotherapy. Despite ongoing mood fluctuations, she learned to deal with her illness sufficiently that, in addition to working, she was able to develop a meaningful relationship leading to marriage and motherhood. During her courtship with her fiancé, she asked for a number of couples sessions to help her fiancé understand her illness and to help them negotiate more effective ways of meeting each other's needs.

In this case the psychiatrist performed the roles of a pharmacotherapist, psychotherapist, and family therapist. The patient and all family members appeared comfortable with and appreciative of having one person provide this comprehensive "family care."

Jim S

Jim S, a 42-year-old married salesman with two sons, presented with a 6-month history of worsening depression and uncertainty about continuing his marriage of 15 years. He had one previous episode of depression that resolved with psychotherapy over an 8-month period. He came for the initial evaluation together with his wife. In addition to confirming the presence of a major depressive disorder, it was clear that there were significant marital problems. Both the patient and his wife wanted to work on improving their marriage. Jim was started on sertraline 50 mg/day, a family evaluation was undertaken, and the decision was made to proceed with couples therapy. During the course of the therapy, it became evident that Jim's wife had difficulty identifying and asserting her own needs. It was agreed she would benefit from individual therapy. Because of the psychiatrist's time constraints, she was referred to a psychologist to work on her individual issues. Jim was seen by the psychiatrist for a few individual sessions, but he preferred to work on his problems in the context of the marital therapy. Over the following few months, Jim's depression resolved and the couple made significant progress in consolidating their relationship. In this case, the psychiatrist functioned mainly as a family therapist and a pharmacotherapist for Jim.

David D

David D, a 56-year-old executive married for 30 years with three adult children, presented with agitation, anxiety, and sadness secondary to the potential breakup of his marriage. His wife was increasingly unhappy in the marriage and talking about leaving him. She in turn was in individual psychotherapy working on deciding what she wanted from life. The psychiatrist's initial evaluation determined that David was not clinically depressed but undergoing an adjustment reaction to the impending threat of losing his wife and family. David and his wife asked to be seen together to determine if the marriage was salvageable. The psychiatrist felt that David would benefit from individual therapy to help him to become more confident asserting his needs and deal with unresolved issues from his family of origin. He referred David to a psychotherapist, deciding not to treat David himself, given that his wife had her own psychotherapist and he felt it would be better for David to have a comparable independent support system. Over time, David's anxiety and agitation diminished and significant progress was made, which improved the marital relationship. In this case, the psychiatrist functioned mainly as a family therapist.

Implementing Integrated Treatment

It is appropriate for a psychiatrist to choose the range of therapies that he or she wants to provide if the decisions are acceptable to the patient and his or her significant others and the psychiatrist is comfortable with these multiple roles. In this situation the psychiatrist has to remain particularly careful about confidentiality and boundaries. Patients and families become more comfortable having one therapist provide multiple therapies when they understand the rationale for doing so. The psychiatrist needs to explain his or her approach as focusing on the presenting problems as well as on the broader context in which these problems exist. The psychiatrist needs to be identified not only as the patient's therapist but also as the professional interested in the welfare and well-being of both the patient and his or her significant others. The patient and family members must understand the rationale for combining different modalities of treatment. When the psychiatrist provides integrated care, there is an inherent efficiency although the practice can be challenging.

Conclusion

This chapter has reviewed the current literature on combined and integrated treatment and has provided case examples illustrating practical points. Clinicians will have to decide which approach most suits the needs of their patients, which approach they are most expert in providing, and what is practical given fiscal realities and the availability of trained therapists.

We have demonstrated in this chapter that it is possible, appropriate, and often desirable for a psychiatrist to provide pharmacotherapy, individual therapy, and family therapy to the same patient. Unfortunately, current practice patterns are moving in the direction of fragmenting treatment among psychiatrists, psychologists, and family therapists. Some professional organizations (e.g., the American Psychological Association) have explicit rules restricting a therapist from providing individual and family therapy to the same patient.

As in any clinical situation, it is critical that the therapist be well trained, proficient in delivering care, able to maintain clear boundaries, and conscientiously adherent to the principle of doing no harm. With those injunctions in mind, the psychiatrist is in a unique position to provide truly integrated biopsychosocial care.

References

1. Gabbard G, Kay J: The fate of integrated treatment: whatever happened to the biopsychosocial psychiatrist? Am J Psychiatry 158:1956–1963, 2001
2. Friedman MA, Detweiler-Bedell JB, Leventhal HE, et al: Combined psychotherapy and pharmacotherapy for the treatment of major depressive disorder. Clin Psychol Sci Prac 11:47–68, 2004
3. Bowers WA: Treatment of depressed inpatients: cognitive therapy plus medication, relaxation plus medication, and medication alone. Br J Psychiatry 156:73–78, 1990
4. Paykel ES, Scott JD, Teasdale JD: Prevention of relapse in residual depression by cognitive therapy: a controlled trial. Arch Gen Psychiatry 56:829–835, 1999
5. Reynolds CF III, Frank E, Perel JM: Nortriptyline and interpersonal psychotherapy as maintenance therapies for recurrent major depression: a randomized controlled trial in patients older than 59 years. JAMA 281:39–45, 1999
6. Teasdale JD, Segel ZV, William JM: Prevention of relapse/recurrence in major depression by mindfulness-based cognitive therapy. J Consult Clin Psychol 68:615–623, 2000
7. Weissman MM, Klerman GL, Paykel E, et al: Treatment effects on the social adjustment of depressed patients. Arch Gen Psychiatry 30:771–778, 1974
8. Hellerstein DJ, Little SA, Samstag LW: Adding group psychotherapy to medication treatment in dysthymias: a randomized prospective pilot study. J Psychother Pract Res 10:93–103, 2001
9. Otto MW, Smits JAJ, Reese HE: Combined psychotherapy and pharmacotherapy for mood and anxiety disorders in adults: review and analyses. Clin Psychol Sci Prac 12:72–86, 2005
10. Thase ME: What role do atypical antipsychotic drugs have in treatment-resistant depression? J Clin Psychiatry 63:95–103, 2002
11. Leff J, Vearnals S, Wolff G, et al: The London Depression Intervention Trial: randomized controlled trial of antidepressants v. couple therapy in the treatment and maintenance of people with depression living with a partner: clinical outcome and costs. Br J Psychiatry 177:95–100, 2000

12. Miklowitz DJ, Johnson SL: The psychopathology and treatment of bipolar disorder. Ann Rev Clin Psychol 2:199–235, 2006

13. Hogarty GE, Kornblith SJ, Greenwald D, et al: Three-year trials of personal therapy among schizophrenic patients living with or independent of family, I: description of study and effects on relapse rates. Am J Psychiatry 154:1504–1513, 1997

14. Mavissakalian MR: Combined behavior and pharmacological treatment of anxiety disorders, in American Psychiatric Press Review of Psychiatry, Vol. 12. Edited by Oldham JM, Riba MB, Tasman A. Washington, DC, American Psychiatric Press, 1993, pp 565–584

15. Miller IW, Norman WH, Keitner GI: Cognitive-behavioral treatment of depressed inpatients: six- and twelve-month follow-up. Am J Psychiatry 146:1274–1279, 1989

16. Thase ME, Greenhouse JB, Frank E: Treatment of major depression with psychotherapy or psychotherapy-pharmacotherapy combinations. Arch Gen Psychiatry 54:1009–1015, 1997

17. Prusoff BA, Weissman MM, Klerman GL, et al: Research diagnostic criteria subtypes of depression: their role as predictors of differential response to psychotherapy and drug treatment. Arch Gen Psychiatry 37:796–801, 1980

18. Keller MB, McCullough JP, Klein DN: A comparison of nefazodone, the cognitive behavioral-analysis system of psychotherapy, and their combination for the treatment of chronic depression. N Engl J Med 342:1462–1470, 2000

19. Thase M, Rush AJ: When at first you don't succeed: sequential strategies for antidepressant nonresponders. J Clin Psychiatry 58 (suppl 13):23–29, 1997

20. Fava GA, Grandi S, Zielesny M: Cognitive behavioral treatment of residual symptoms in primary major depressive disorder. Am J Psychiatry 151:1295–1299, 1994

21. Goldapple K, Segal Z, Garson C: Modulation of cortical-limbic pathways in major depression: treatment-specific effects of cognitive behavior therapy. Arch Gen Psychiatry 61:34–41, 2004

22. Mayberg HS: Modulating limbic-cortical circuits in depression: targets of antidepressant treatments. Sem Clin Neuropsychiatry 7:255–268, 2002

23. Castren E: Is mood chemistry? Nat Rev Neurosci 6:241–246, 2005

24. Basco MR, Rush AJ: Compliance with pharmacotherapy in mood disorders. Psychiatr Ann 25:269–279, 1995

25. de Jonghe F, Kool S, van Aalst G: Combining psychotherapy and antidepressants in the treatment of depression. J Affect Dis 64:217–299, 2001

26. Vergouwen AC, Bakker A, Katon WJ: Improving adherence to antidepressants: a systematic review of interventions. J Clin Psychiatry 64:1415–1420, 2003

27. Seligman ME: The effectiveness of psychotherapy: the Consumer Reports study. Am Psychol 50:965–974, 1995

28. Krupnick JL, Sotsky SM, Simmens S: The role of the therapeutic alliance in psychotherapy and pharmacotherapy outcome: findings in the National Institute of Mental Health Treatment of Depression Collaborative Research Program. J Consult Clin Psychol 64:532–539, 1996

29. Fava GA, Ruini C, Rafanelli C: Sequential treatment of mood and anxiety disorders. J Clin Psychiatry 66:1392–1400, 2005

30. Buckley PF, Brown ES: Prevalence and consequences of dual diagnosis. J Clin Psychiatry 67:e01, 2006

31. Minkoff K, Cline CA: Changing the world: the design and implementation of comprehensive continuous integrated systems of care for individuals with co-occurring disorders. Psychiatr Clin North Am 27:727–743, 2004

32. Mangrum LF, Spence RT, Lopez M: Integrated versus parallel treatment of co-occurring psychiatric and substance use disorders. J Subst Abuse Treat 30:79–84, 2006

33. Oxman TE, Schulberg HC, Greenberg RI, et al: A fidelity measure for integrated management of depression in primary care. Med Care 44:1030–1037, 2006

34. Schotte CKW, Van Den Bossche B, De Doncker D, et al: A biopsychosocial model as a guide for psychoeducation and treatment of depression. Depress Anxiety 23:312–324, 2006

35. Bauer MS, McBride L, Williford WG, et al: Collaborative care for bipolar disorder, Part II: impact on clinical outcome, function, and costs. Psychiatr Serv 57:937–945, 2006

36. Goldman W, McCulloch J, Cuffel B, et al: Outpatient utilization patterns of integrated and split psychotherapy and pharmacotherapy for depression. Psychiatr Serv 49:477–482, 1998

37. Glick ID: Combining pharmacotherapy with psychotherapeutic management: guidelines for integration. J Clin Psychiatry 67:1645–1646, 2006

38. Dewan M: Are psychiatrists cost-effective? An analysis of integrated versus split treatment. Am J Psychiatry 156:324–326, 1999

39. Mintz DL, Belnap BA, Katon WJ: What is psychodynamic psychopharmacology? An approach to psychopharmacologic treatment resistance. J Am Acad Psychoanal 34:581–601, 2006

11

Family Interventions With Specific Disorders

- Adjunctive family interventions are helpful in the treatment of many psychiatric disorders.
- The experience of each family and the family's understanding of the illness need to be individually assessed.
- Common themes recur with specific disorders requiring a specific knowledge base.

This chapter describes the application of family research to clinical practice. As noted in Chapter 3, there is good evidence to show the effect of a variety of disorders on the functioning of families and the effect of family functioning on the course of a disorder. Studies also show the efficacy of including family interventions in the management of several psychiatric disorders. The findings from these studies suggest ways of approaching families that are helpful for specific disorders.

No studies suggest that specific approaches for dealing with specific issues are of benefit for a particular family with a given psychiatric disorder; rather, results from the various studies provide a guide and framework but do not provide a prescription. Each family needs to be assessed individually to determine what impact the particular disorder has on its functioning and how that functioning is influencing the course of the disorder.

This chapter uses the Problem-Centered Systems Therapy of the Family (PCSTF) to provide a framework for the specific evaluation of the family while incorporating suggestions for managing particular disorders from available research. The PCSTF is designed to evaluate specific problems that a given family presents while also requiring the therapist to complete a comprehensive evaluation. The family and therapist then come to a mutual agreement about the family's specific problems and a plan of action on how to bring about change that is meaningful to all family members. This chapter illustrates these concepts through case examples.

Schizophrenia

Acute Phase

A patient with abnormal beliefs or odd behavior may be showing signs of schizophrenia and a family member may ask, is it schizophrenia? Or if one's father has schizophrenia, one may ask, should I worry about him? These are the "good" cases, in which the family is involved and asks questions. What should the psychiatrist say and do? The impact of the first episode of schizophrenia is different for the family because the family members do not have prior experience with psychosis, the acuteness of the episode is more mystifying, and there is often diagnostic ambiguity. As a result, psychoeducation cannot be as specific as for the family intervention in chronic schizophrenia described in earlier chapters.

Some work on early intervention programs involving high-risk patients provide guidance for psychiatrists. Guidelines offered by Jean Addington and colleagues from the Calgary Early Intervention Program can be followed if no early intervention programs exist in the area (1). Goals at this stage are to maximize the adaptive functioning of the family; minimize the disruption to family life caused by the first episode; minimize the risk of long-term grief, stress, and burden experienced by the family; aid the family to understand the impact of psychosis on the family system and on individual family members; and understand the interaction between family and course of illness. The program uses four stages to plan services for families: managing the crisis, initial stabilization and facilitating recovery, consolidating the gains, and prolonged recovery.

The first stage involves managing the acute crisis of the first psychotic episode and engaging the client and family. This can occur in multiple settings: inpatient unit, home with a mobile team, or outpatient clinic. A detailed collateral history and needs assessment is gathered from the family. Families are given support and assistance to manage the crisis and offered an initial explanatory model of psychosis. At this stage, families who have difficulty facilitating the recovery efforts of their relative or who appear to be managing poorly are identified and offered help from a family therapist. Individual family treatment during this stage consists primarily of frequent contact with workers who offer high levels of support. Specifically, families are offered practical and emotional assistance to minimize the impact of the trauma. Messages about psychosis and its treatment are repeated and conveyed clearly. Education is provided about the role the family can expect to take in the treatment of their ill family member.

The second stage focuses on stabilizing the patient and family and facilitating recovery. The goals are to continue to assess family functioning, consolidate the therapeutic alliance, and increase the family's knowledge of psychosis, including signs of relapse. A related goal is to ensure that families at high risk and those with sustained patterns of dysfunction receive specialized family care.

Family intervention in early schizophrenia

- **Stage 1:** Managing the crisis. Engage the family; provide support, assistance, explanation of psychosis; minimize impact of trauma; provide education

- **Stage 2:** Initial stabilization and facilitating recovery. Assess family functioning, consolidate alliance, and increase family's knowledge

- **Stage 3:** Consolidating the gains. Family and patient incorporate gains from previous stages into day-to-day practices, are taught how to manage relapse, adjust expectations, and maintain psychological well-being

- **Stage 4:** Prolonged recovery. Step down to routine care. Change family's expectations, adapt to less-than-full recovery, develop consensus about prognosis, manage feelings of grief and loss

The third stage focuses on consolidating the gains from the earlier stages. The family and patient learn to incorporate knowledge learned in previous stages into day-to-day practices. Both family and patient are taught to manage relapse risk. Families work on readjusting expectations and maintaining psychological well-being.

The final stage of the recovery model steps the family down to routine care. Goals focus on changing expectations of the family, adapting to less than a full recovery, and developing consensus regarding prognosis for the patient. Family intervention may be needed to help manage feelings of grief and loss.

Using the PCSTF, an individual psychiatrist can incorporate the stages of this model. After the initial assessment, the problem list is drawn up and agreed to. In the process of working through the problem list, the psychiatrist can provide frequent short contacts and written information about psychosis, helping to identify family dysfunction as the family learns to adjust to the illness. Meeting with the patient and family to discuss and manage relapse and to help with adjustment of expectations can also occur. Prior to termination, the psychiatrist can work with the family on agreeing to a prognosis and expected outcome before stepping the patient down to routine care.

Chronic Phase

The standard of care in chronic schizophrenia includes the provision of family psychoeducational groups, as described by McFarlane and colleagues (2) and articulated in the American Psychiatric Association Practice Guidelines (3). If the patient and family do not have access to one of these groups, what can be done? Several studies show that less intense support or education does have benefit. The psychiatrist or another member of the team can initiate an educational or support group or refer the patient and family to a community-based group run by the National Alliance on Mental Illness (NAMI).

Outpatients with schizophrenia in a large community mental health center who received psychoeducational multiple-family group treatment had a lower rate of psychiatric hospitalization compared with patients who received standard care (4). The 2-year multiple-family intervention consisted of weekly group sessions designed to educate patients and family members about the biological basis of mental illness and treatment, improve illness management and coping skills, and provide social support. Group sessions were conducted by two clinicians using a standardized protocol. Each multiple-family group included five to eight families and patients. Implementation of multiple-family group treatment in a capitated community mental health setting improved hospitalization outcomes without increasing overall volume of outpatient mental health services. With some support, this program could be implemented in most mental health centers.

Family intervention in chronic schizophrenia: McFarlane's model

---

- Coordinate care with all providers
- Attend to social needs of family
- Provide optimal medication management
- Listen to families and treat them as equal partners in treatment planning and delivery
- Explore family members' expectations of treatment and for the patient
- Assess family's strengths and limitations in being able to support the patient
- Help resolve family conflict
- Address feelings of loss
- Provide relevant information at appropriate times
- Provide explicit crisis plan
- Improve communication and problem solving
- Encourage family to expand social network
- Be flexible in meeting the family's needs

A peer-led support group for families also can improve patient and family outcome (5). Families were randomly assigned to one of three groups (mutual support, psychoeducation, and standard care), and interventions were delivered at two psychiatric outpatient clinics over a 6-month period. The mutual support and psychoeducation interventions consisted of 12 group sessions every 2 weeks, each lasting 2 hours. The mutual support group was peer-led and designed to provide information, emotional support, and coping skills. The psychoeducation group was a professional-led group designed to educate families about the biological basis of schizophrenia and treatment and to improve illness management and coping skills. All groups received routine psychiatric outpatient care during the intervention. The mutual support intervention was associated with greater improvements in patients' functioning and rehospitalization and stable use of mental health services over the follow-up period compared with the other two interventions.

A curriculum for training peer moderators has been developed (6). Peer moderators are trained to conduct eight 1-hour sessions (warmup, symptoms, diagnosis, causes, medication, psychosocial therapy, warning signs, coping with schizophrenia) with 6–10 patients per group. The feasibility of the curriculum was evaluated via a pilot study of seven peer groups with two peer moderators. On the whole, peer-moderated groups worked well. Knowledge of illness increased significantly and concept of illness changed significantly in three subscales: trust in physician and trust in medication increased, and negative treatment expectations decreased. Subjective assessments of peer moderators by patients were positive. Peer-to-peer psychoeducation in schizophrenia may be comparable with professional psychoeducation with regard to short-term outcomes. In mental health centers, it may be possible to encourage family members to set up their own support groups and provide training, space, and educational material.

If no resources are available within the clinic, then the patient and family can be referred to NAMI. A well-established peer-to-peer program run by NAMI is the Family-to-Family Education Program. It consists of a 12-week course for family members of adults with serious mental illness, taught by peers and sponsored by NAMI. This program has been disseminated throughout most of the United States and Puerto Rico and is also available with some support groups in Mexico and Canada (Ontario and British Columbia). Families who have attended have reduced subjective burden, increased empowerment, improved knowledge about mental illness, gained better understanding of the mental health system, and improved self-care (7).

For the psychiatrist, working with a patient with chronic schizophrenia and his or her family can be a rewarding experience. The family is usually grateful to be asked into the treatment setting, and the patient benefits from a more functional family environment that comes with an improved family understanding of the illness. Using the PCSTF, the psychiatrist completes an assessment. Questions related to affective responsiveness and affective involvement are presented in this assessment with the knowledge and understanding that the patient with chronic schizophrenia will be less involved and may experience increased symptoms with intense family affect. During this assessment, the psychiatrist can educate the family about schizophrenia and support the family in maintaining an emotional environment that is of low intensity. If the family is highly emotionally expressive with high hostility, education can be given about deleterious effects on patient outcome. It would also be appropriate to provide patients and families with educational literature at this time. Educational deficits about schizophrenia would therefore be a priority on the problem list and one of the main foci of treatment.

Other issues frequently brought up by families with a chronic schizophrenic member include family involvement in treatment, medication compliance, and daily schedules at home. It is often important for the patient to have a meaningful role in the family or in the community. These issues can be identified and placed on the problem list.

Schizophrenia Case Example

Sadie, a 26-year-old woman who lived with her parents and worked part time in a department store, was admitted with her second episode of psychosis. She had been on fluphenazine 10 mg for 5 years with stability, but she recently had a change in insurance and went to a new psychiatrist who prescribed her an atypical antipsychotic. Unfortunately, she decompensated and was hospitalized. The patient adamantly refused to have her parents involved, stating they had abused her when she was a child and in fact were instruments of the devil, who was responsible for her becoming psychotic. After her fluphenazine was reestablished, she slowly retreated from this position but was clearly anxious and apprehensive whenever her parents visited her.

The psychiatrist understood that a family assessment would be needed to get a clear understanding of Sadie's situation, despite her reluctance to have her parents included in her treatment. With her permission, the psychiatrist first sat with Sadie and her family when they came for visits, after which she agreed to participate in several short meetings "to understand better how things are at home." The psychiatrist decided to do an assessment in short stages, because the patient's tolerance for sitting with her parents was poor. A full assessment was completed over several meetings. The parents were shocked to hear Sadie's accusations of abuse and delusions about the devil pressing down on her body at night. While the patient and family were passively willing to meet and to agree on the assessment, the psychiatrist had to be very active and do much of the work.

Problem solving: The family generally worked well together on both affective and instrumental problems. The family brought Sadie quickly to the hospital when she decompensated.

Communication: This was generally good except when Sadie became ill.

Role allocation: The family had several appropriate family rituals such as eating the evening meal together most evenings. There were no financial problems, and each member was generally satisfied with the division of household chores, work, and future life goals.

Affective responsiveness: The parents were worried about Sadie's current mental status as well as her future stability and care. The family generally maintained a quiet, calm home.

Affective involvement: When Sadie was well, her parents enjoyed a mutually supportive relationship with friends and outside activities. When Sadie became ill, they focused on her care and dropped outside activities. They agreed it was important to return to these when Sadie became stable. Sadie and her mother went shopping together. Sadie and her father would play cards together. When she was well, Sadie also had friends with whom she went out to dinner and to movies.

Behavior control: There were no current significant issues identified. The formulation presented to the family conveyed that the family functioned well normally but became acutely destabilized when Sadie got ill. The psychiatrist indicated that the focus of family treatment was to get Sadie well and the family back to its prior level of good functioning. Sadie indicated that she also wished to move out and live on her own. The problem list was as follows:

1. Sadie's illness required her to take fluphenazine and to find a psychiatrist who would respect her wishes regarding this medication.
2. The family, including Sadie, was very distressed at her hospitalization and wanted to ensure it never happened again. All agreed to work hard to re-establish the family's prior level of functioning.
3. Her parents refuted Sadie's claims of childhood abuse.
4. Sadie would work to become independent of her parents.

The strengths of this family were that they cared deeply about each other, were uncritical of each other, and were respectful of each other's opinions. They valued time together and were invested in each other's hobbies and interests. They were financially stable. The first two problems on the list were easily addressed, and the psychiatrist helped the family negotiate who would find the psychiatrist and how to help Sadie come to terms with her hospitalization. Problem 3 was insolvable because the patient insisted that abuse had taken place and the parents denied it. The psychiatrist stated that if they were going to live together, continued disagreement and fighting would severely affect the health of all concerned. They all agreed to not discuss this issue further. The first step in Sadie's independence was returning to work, while both parents agreed to help transport her to interviews and help her fill out application forms.

This family's strengths allowed them to work together for the benefit of the patient. It was impossible to assess the truth of Sadie's claim of childhood abuse, but it was possible to work with her and the family toward her future independence. The assessment took place over three short interviews, and the treatment occurred in two short follow-up meetings. This example shows how it is possible to be flexible with scheduling and the importance of being respectful of both the recovering patient and her family despite a deep and likely irreconcilable family rift.

Bipolar Disorder

In bipolar disorder, as in other disorders, stresses can act on vulnerable individuals to precipitate illness. The first episode of bipolar disorder is often precipitated by a stressful life event (8). A range of family factors are implicated in the onset and course of bipolar disorders. These include dysfunctional early relationships with parents, communication deviance, high expressed emotion in families, family conflict, and lack of social support (9).

Coping with bipolar disorder is particularly difficult for families because of the chronic remitting and relapsing nature of the illness. Generally, only one-third of patients have a persistently good course, whereas two-thirds have either some form of ongoing residual symptoms or a fluctuating course with multiple episodes over time (10). Family members describe losses pertaining to hopes, dreams, and expectations and grieve for what might have been. Significant adjustments may need to be made, possibly decreasing work hours or taking time off during episodes of illness, which can lead to financial stress (11).

Responses to the illness vary depending on the phase of the disorder. Patients experiencing depression and mania exhibit different challenging symptoms. Family responses depend on the role of the patient in the family and whether this is a first episode or an ongoing recurrent pattern. Families live with uncertainty about acute disruptions, including potentially violent and risky behavior and not knowing when the next episode may strike.

Family members can also mitigate the impact of the illness. Resilient families are characterized by mutual support, clear and direct communication, collaborative problem solving, the maintenance of a strong family structure, and the establishment of good emotional relatedness (12). The quality of the marital relationship is a stress modifier such that a good relationship moderates the effects of stressors. Families may hinder a patient's recovery by pressuring the patient to resume premorbid responsibilities prematurely. Family members' fear and anxiety may exacerbate the patient's concerns, leading to continued disruption in social and marital roles. Conversely, a family may contribute positively to the patient's improvement by assisting with medication and treatment compliance, monitoring symptoms and side effects, helping with the logistical issues of accessing health care, sharing role responsibilities, and promoting more regular and structured lifestyles. Family members can often recognize both prodromal and residual symptoms of the illness and can be helpful in identifying the need for early interventions and monitoring the continuation of treatment even when the acute episode appears to have subsided (13).

Despite optimal pharmacotherapy, relapse is almost inevitable for patients with bipolar disorder. Adjunctive psychosocial treatments including family therapy delay the time to relapse and help avoid hospitalization (see Chapter 3). Family interventions, while not affecting the patient's symptomatic status in any major way, do make significant differences for families. Family interventions clearly improve the family's knowledge and understanding of the illness and also lead to a lessened sense of isolation and a decrease in the family's perception of illness burden.

Family intervention in bipolar disorder

- Improve problem-solving skills and communications
- Decrease levels of criticism within the family
- Develop and improve coping skills
- Develop strategies for dealing with relapses

As with other psychiatric disorders, each family's situation, coping skills, feelings of burden, and available resources differ. Each family needs to be individually assessed to determine their needs and capabilities. This can be done through the framework of the PCSTF (see Chapter 9). Specific areas related to the management of bipolar disorder focus on improving problem-solving skills and communications, decreasing levels of criticism within the family, developing and improving coping skills, and developing strategies for dealing with relapses. These improved skills, in conjunction with education that empowers the family, can buffer patient and family members against the difficulties created by the fluctuating course of the illness.

Bipolar Disorder Case Example

Mr. B, a 35-year-old single mortgage loan salesman, was hospitalized for a manic episode. He was brought from the airport by the police because of disruptive behaviors. He had gone on a traveling and spending spree following 10 days of sleeplessness, increased energy, pressured speech, grandiosity, and irritability. He had no insight into his illness and was outraged at being hospitalized.

Mr. B had been living with his parents for the past 6 months subsequent to losing his job when his mortgage company went bankrupt. He was looking for new work and taking night courses at a local college. He had never been married. He had one previous manic episode in his 20s and a number of depressions that had responded to pharmacological treatment in the past. He had stopped all of his medications 4 years prior to the current episode. He did not accept that he had a chronic remitting and relapsing illness.

During his hospitalization he was treated with divalproex 750 mg two times per day and risperidone 2 mg at bedtime. A family meeting was held during which both parents were very defensive about their son's behavior and lack of compliance with long-term prophylactic pharmacological treatment. They minimized the severity of his illness and need for hospitalization. They were also resistant to learning more about bipolar disorder and its long-term management, and anxious to protect and please their son and to not look too closely at the stresses that may have contributed to precipitating his current episode.

Once the patient was stabilized, he was discharged to follow-up care but was noncompliant. He was readmitted to the hospital 2 weeks later, once again in a full-blown manic episode. By this time, the parents were more amenable to trying to understand the nature of their son's illness and the role that they might play in helping him deal with it more effectively.

During the second family meeting, the psychiatrist once again oriented the family to the goals of the meeting. He emphasized again his habit of meeting with the families of all his patients to minimize the perception that they were in any way being blamed for their son's difficulties. He encouraged them to outline problems as they saw them and to ask questions about the illness and its longer-term management. The patient and parents then proceeded to identify problems. Both parents expressed concern about their son's current lack of employment, his unstructured lifestyle, tendency to keep irregular hours, and lack of follow-up with prescribed treatment. The patient also expressed frustration with having to live at home and not being able to find a new job. He acknowledged he was having difficulty accepting the chronicity of his illness. He felt infantilized by his parents yet at the same time demanded that they continue to look after him.

The psychiatrist then reviewed the family's overall functioning along with the dimensions of family functioning as outlined in the McMaster Model. Overall, the family's functioning was good except for a few areas. They had difficulty solving problems because they were reluctant to look at information that they were uncomfortable with. They were somewhat overinvolved with their son, leading to an accommodation to his illness behavior rather than helping him set a more reality-based framework. They had few expectations in terms of his contributing to the daily running of their home. They were also reluctant to establish and hold to clear expectations about responsibilities in continuing to live with them.

The psychiatrist presented his opinion that the patient was suffering from bipolar disorder that was based on a genetic vulnerability, possibly precipitated by the distress of having lost his job, being unable to find a new job, the lack of regularity and routine in his life, and his noncompliance with long-term outpatient follow-up care. The psychiatrist also suggested that the parents may have been overprotective and overaccommodating to their son, with the result that he was now having difficulty regulating himself.

The parents and patient agreed with this formulation, which represented information that they had provided. The psychiatrist asked the family members what they wanted to do about the agreed-upon problems. They felt that they needed to learn more about bipolar disorder and its treatment and long-term course. They agreed on the importance of ensuring compliance with pharmacological and psychosocial treatments. The parents decided to set clearer expectations about responsibilities in the running of the home and about regularity in their son's life (e.g., meal and sleep times). They also wanted to feel more comfortable discussing problems as they came up, without feeling that they were going to upset their son.

After discharge from the hospital, the patient continued on prophylactic divalproex and outpatient psychotherapy to help him come to terms with the nature of his illness and to provide support while he recovered from his acute episode and struggled to find new employment. The family met with the psychiatrist on an outpatient basis for two sessions to ensure that they were working toward their chosen goals. During that time, the psychiatrist also provided them with more information about bipolar disorder and referred them to a local self-help group for continued support and an opportunity to learn from others about managing bipolar disorders.

Major Depression

Depressive disorders encompass a wide range of conditions with varying degrees of severity and dysfunction. These disorders are truly biopsychosocial in their etiology. Most depressions are presumed to result from a confluence of psychological and social stressors acting on a biologically vulnerable person. The relative contributions of biological, psychological, and social factors are different for each patient. An understanding of the patient and the interventions that are likely to be effective for that patient need to be individually assessed.

Family intervention in major depression

- Improve communication
- Improve family support
- Clarify family roles
- Provide information about depression, course of illness, and available treatments
- Reduce blame, hostility, and criticism
- Set realistic goals that accompany recovery of functioning

The role of the family in the etiology and course of depression has been extensively studied (14, 15, 16). Family stresses that are associated with the development of depression include parental psychopathology, parental loss, marital discord, separation and divorce, family violence, abuse, neglect, social adversity, and economic hardship (15). The level of expressed emotion (EE) in a family has a significant impact on the course of the depressive illness, with patients from high EE families relapsing at a lower level of criticism than patients with schizophrenia (17).

As with other disorders, the cause-and-effect nature of the relationship between depression and family dysfunction is most likely circular. Dysfunctional families' interactional styles may potentiate the development of a depressive episode, but the presence of depression in a family member may also contribute significantly to family dysfunction. It is helpful to try to determine whether the family dysfunction predated or followed the onset of the depressive episode. If problems in the family appear to be a result of the depressive episode, the family intervention that may be most helpful is likely to be different than in a situation in which family disturbances were a chronic background to the depression. If the family stresses are a function of difficulties coping with the depressive episode, the treatment of the depression, along with support and education for the family, may be sufficient to ensure that the family will return to its premorbid normal level of functioning. A family with chronic patterns of dysfunction needs comprehensive family assessment and treatment.

There is no "typical" pattern of family dysfunction unique to patients with depression. Each family attempts to cope with the reality of its ill member in ways that are unique to the individuals and circumstances that make up that family constellation. The ways in which families deal with the depression have a significant impact on the duration of the depressive episode, the likelihood of recovery, and recurrence (18).

A number of studies have attempted to evaluate the effectiveness of couples/marital treatment for depression (10, 19). In general, the evidence suggests that family therapy is a useful adjunct to pharmacotherapy for patients with depression, particularly when the depression is severe or when the depressive episode evolves in the presence of marital/family distress. Marital therapy may be comparable with cognitive therapy in relieving symptoms of depression, but marital therapy may be more effective in improving marital satisfaction, particularly when marital distress is part of the clinical presentation.

Particular foci of family interventions should be on improving the communications, support, and fulfillment of parental roles. It is important to provide information about the nature of depression, available treatments, and the likely course of illness. The goal is to reduce blame and the accompanying hostility and criticism toward the patient for social withdrawal, negativity, seeming dependence, and apparent hopelessness and helplessness. With a better understanding of the nature of the illness, the realistic capabilities of the patient can be determined and family members can support the patient in the fulfillment of those objectives that are within their capacity to manage. Goals can include direct and clear communication of concerns, a gradually increasing and fuller involvement in necessary family roles, and gradually increasing participation in activities outside of the home, along with greater levels of physical activity.

The challenge to the therapist is to determine the particular goals of any given family and the obstacles that may be preventing them from achieving those goals. This formulation is most likely to be successful through meeting with all the family members available so that different perspectives on the problem can be elicited and ways the family understands and has tried to deal with the problem can be determined. This process of assessment and clarification of the family's difficulties can be of significant therapeutic value in and of itself as it may provide an opportunity for the family to hear each other's concerns in a safe environment in a way that was perhaps not possible up to that point. Families may have been reluctant to express their perspectives to each other for fear of hurting each other's feelings or because of the anger that each may have felt about the burden they have been dealing with.

Once family members have had an opportunity to express themselves and to have their views of the situation validated in a nonjudgmental environment, they are more likely to be able to listen to other family members' perspectives and to work toward adjustments and compromises in the way in which they approach their problems. If those significant others are not directly involved in the process of treatment, bringing about changes in the social environment to more effectively meet the needs not only of the patient but also of significant others involved in their care is less likely to happen.

Major Depression Case Example

Mr. D, a 52-year-old teacher, was referred by his wife, a nurse, for evaluation of depressive symptoms. He had been experiencing poor sleep, poor appetite, anxiety, poor concentration, sadness, and low energy. He had been having increasing difficulties functioning at work. He had two previous depressive episodes but had been symptom free for the past 10 years. He was thinking of separating from his wife of 26 years but was unable to decide what to do.

Upon obtaining the referral, the psychiatrist asked to see Mr. and Mrs. D for an initial evaluation. Mr. D had no comorbid medical or substance abuse problems. He met criteria for major depression and was started on sertraline 50 mg/day. The evaluation also identified significant marital problems that had predated the depression and seemed to have worsened since the second of their two children left home 2 years ago. At the conclusion of the initial evaluation, Mr. and Mrs. D decided they wanted to continue seeing the psychiatrist to help determine the viability of their marriage simultaneously with Mr. D's depression being treated, feeling that his inability to resolve his ambivalence about the marriage was a significant contributor to his depression. Mr. D declined concurrent individual therapy.

During the subsequent family evaluation, the psychiatrist outlined the goal of that session to have the couple identify their problems. Mr. D complained that he felt emotionally distant from his wife, was bored with their relationship, was frustrated by feeling increasingly inadequate at work in relation to his younger and more ambitious colleagues, and could not see how any of this could be changed. Mrs. D felt her husband did not share his feelings with her, tended to go his own way without involving her, put her down in the social settings, and was sexually unresponsive to her.

The psychiatrist then evaluated their functioning as a couple along the family dimensions outlined in the McMaster Model. He found that Mr. D had great difficulty communicating about emotions, while Mrs. D wanted to talk about emotional issues to a degree that made Mr. D uncomfortable. They were able to deal with instrumental but not affective problems and were affectively disconnected from each other. Role allocation was acceptable to both, but Mr. D tended to leave household management to his wife. Mr. D had a habit of not letting his wife know his whereabouts even when she asked to be informed.

The psychiatrist shared his formulation with the couple, suggesting Mr. D's depression was likely the result of multiple factors. Mr. D had a biological vulnerability to depression as evidenced by his previous episodes and family history of depression. A number of current stresses contributed to the onset of the current episode. Mr. D's stage of life and thoughts about job satisfaction and capabilities weighed heavily on him. He was unhappy with the emotional distance from his wife and his inability to connect to her at a time when he had great need for that connection. He responded by withdrawing and criticizing her, which in turn pushed her further away, leaving him even more isolated. For her part, Mrs. D alternated between frantic efforts to breach her husband's affective barriers and anger and withdrawal when she was unsuccessful. The combination of stresses at work and lack of sufficient support at home in conjunction with his vulnerability to depression likely led to the current episode.

The couple agreed with the formulation and decided they wanted to work on improving their marriage. Mr. D wanted to be able to talk to his wife about his feelings of unease at work, but in a way that was comfortable for him. At the same time, he wanted his wife to not cater to him in all matters but rather to assert herself in a way he had found attractive when they first met. Mrs. D wanted her husband to share his concerns with her more openly. She also wanted him to be less critical and demeaning toward her. She also wanted him to keep her informed more openly about his whereabouts.

Over the next five sessions, there was significant improvement in Mr. D's symptoms of depression as well as his functioning at work. He tolerated an increased dose of sertraline without significant side effects. The couple worked hard at their tasks but found it difficult to equilibrate their different personality styles and level of comfort with emotional issues. With guided practice, Mr. D became more comfortable expressing his vulnerabilities, and as he did so, his wife had less need to intrude past his level of comfort. As Mr. D felt more supported, he criticized his wife less. Their sex life also improved. Mr. D decided that he wanted to continue the marriage. (**For another case example of the impact of depression on the family, watch the DVD.**)

Alcoholism and Substance Abuse Disorders

Behavioral couples therapy (BCT) for married or cohabiting drug-abusing and alcoholic patients results in positive outcomes with 1) fewer days of alcohol and drug use, 2) fewer arrests, 3) fewer alcohol- or drug-related hospitalizations, 4) higher relationship satisfaction, and 5) reduced levels of partner violence at posttreatment and through 12-month follow-up than alcoholic and drug-abusing patients receiving more traditional individual-based treatment (20). To build support for sobriety, BCT includes the spouse with the substance-abusing patient. A daily sobriety contract is drawn up in which the patient states his or her intention not to drink or use drugs that day and the spouse expresses support for the patient's efforts to stay abstinent. If appropriate, daily Antabuse ingestion witnessed by the spouse can also be part of the contract. The spouse records the performance of the daily contract on a calendar provided by the therapist. Both partners agree not to discuss past drinking or fears about future drinking to prevent substance-related conflicts, which can trigger relapse, and to reserve these discussions for therapy sessions.

At the start of each BCT couple session, the therapist reviews the sobriety contract calendar to see how well each spouse has done his or her part. If the sobriety contract includes 12-step meetings or urine drug screens, these are also marked on the calendar and reviewed. The calendar provides an ongoing record of progress that is rewarded verbally at each session. The couple performs the behaviors of their sobriety contract in each session to highlight its importance and lets the therapist observe how the couple carries out the contract. In this way, BCT increases positive feelings, shared activities, and constructive communication because these relationship factors are conducive to sobriety. In "Catch Your Partner Doing Something Nice," each spouse notices and acknowledges one pleasing behavior performed by their partner each day. In the "Caring Day" assignment, each person plans ahead to surprise the spouse with a day when they do special things to show their caring. "Planning and Doing Shared Rewarding Activities" is important because many substance abusers' families have stopped shared activities, which are associated with positive recovery outcomes. Each activity must involve both spouses, either by themselves or with their children or other adults, and can be at or away from home. Teaching communication skills can help the alcoholic patient and spouse deal with stressors in their relationship and in their lives, which may reduce risk of relapse. At the end of weekly BCT sessions, each couple completes a Continuing Recovery Plan that is reviewed at quarterly follow-up visits for an additional 2 years.

Family intervention in alcohol dependence

- Sobriety contract
- "Catch Your Partner Doing Something Nice" assignment
- "Caring Day" assignment
- "Planning and Doing Shared Rewarding Activities" assignment
- Teaching communication skills

If the clinic or physician has concerns about cost, a brief BCT is now available that does not provide the full benefit of BCT as described above but does reduce drinking and improve relational functioning (21). In a survey of substance abuse treatment agencies regarding the use of conjoint treatments (22), the majority of program administrators (85%) indicated they would offer a couples-based intervention to their patients if it was brief, was shown to be effective in reducing substance use and improving other outcomes, and could be readily integrated into existing treatments (e.g., individual and group counseling). Brief BCT meets all of these criteria, although couples with very severe relationship problems and patients with long-standing alcohol dependence may require more intensive treatment.

Providers need not choose between brief BCT and BCT if these interventions are viewed as part of a stepped care treatment model whereby couples entering conjoint treatment receive the less intensive treatment initially. Couples who do not reach their treatment goals in the brief treatment modality are offered further treatment at a higher (i.e., stepped-up) level of intensity. Studies on a stepped care model of couples therapy for alcoholism have yet to be conducted but are an important future research direction.

In the individual psychiatrist's practice, whether an inpatient, partial hospital, or outpatient setting, it is possible to implement the steps of BCT. Inviting the spouse into the evaluation and including the spouse in the diagnostic formulation and then in the treatment planning is beneficial. Once the spouse agrees to be involved, a sobriety contract can be established and behavioral tasks prescribed. If the couple fails to respond or if further relationship difficulties arise, the couple can be referred to a family therapist.

Alcohol Dependence Case Example

Mrs. B, a 64-year-old married female, was brought by the police to the hospital intoxicated and combative. Once she had completed detoxification, a family meeting was convened with her husband and their 30-year-old son. The psychiatrist began by stating that the purpose of the meeting was to gather information about Mrs. B's alcohol history and to assess what role the family might play in her recovery. An assessment was completed during which it was clear that the husband was not fully committed to the marriage.

Problem solving: Generally, the family did well, although in this instance because of Mr. B's absence from the home, Mrs. B's alcohol dependence had escalated unchecked. The son had already decided during the course of the meeting how to rectify this issue, indicating good problem solving on an instrumental level. Affective problem solving remained poor as evidenced by the lack of identification of Mrs. B's difficulties, which had clearly started years before.

A problem list was drawn up:

1. Mrs. B has a serious addiction to alcohol and needs to attend all follow-ups as recommended by her outpatient psychiatrist.
2. As a result of her drinking, her relationship with her husband is severely strained.

3. Mr. B's work schedule takes him out of town too frequently.
4. The son is involved and will attend outpatient care with her and monitor her when her husband is out of town.

Communication: There was little communication between the couple, with the son often being the intermediary. The son indicated his availability and willingness to remain in this role until his mother received treatment.

Role allocation: The son acknowledged that he had taken on a large care-giving role. Mr. B continued to fulfill all instrumental family roles such as bill paying, shopping, and upkeep of their home.

Affective responsiveness: Mrs. B was able to express that her loneliness and lack of employment had been precursors to possible depressive symptoms and alcohol dependence. The psychiatrist had to decide how to make the husband's disconnection explicit in the meeting, asking the husband, "Are you committed to this marriage?" The husband replied in the affirmative and the psychiatrist proceeded, taking him at his word. The patient, recognizing what was being asked, added: "I have driven my husband away and it is my responsibility to stop drinking and try to win him back."

Affective involvement: Mr. B was often away from the house on business, could not supply important details of his wife's mental state during the past year, and in fact deferred many questions to his son. He was affectively disconnected from his wife.

Behavior control: All agreed that alcohol was the major destabilizing factor and no significant issues existed in its absence. The son thought he might stay with his mother whenever the father was out of town in order to monitor her.

In treatment, the family signed a sobriety contract and worked out a schedule whereby either the husband or the son could monitor and take the daily pledge with the patient. In this way, the behavioral aspects needed for recovery were put into place. No attempt was made to specifically treat the marital conflict, as it was considered too severe because of the husband's lack of involvement. This assessment can of course be revisited as treatment progresses. This case illustrates the important work that can be done even in the presence of severe marital difficulties. Assessment was key to identifying the husband's lack of involvement and the son's willingness to help out. Assessment facilitated behavioral treatment to be put into place.

Anxiety Disorders

Most family research on anxiety disorders has focused on patients and families with panic disorders, with or without agoraphobia, and on obsessive-compulsive disorders (23).

Panic Disorder With Agoraphobia

There are a variety of theories about the etiology of panic disorder. Cognitive-behavioral theorists postulate that anxiety arises from faulty evaluation of and misattribution of internal and external stimuli (24). Interpersonal theorists (25) suggest that agoraphobia is related to problems differentiating from families of origin. Psychodynamic theorists understand panic to be the result of difficulties in the infant-mother relationship leading to inability on the child's part to soothe him- or herself in later life (26). Other theories focus on receptor hypersensitivity (27), leading to dysregulation of the hypothalamic-pituitary-adrenal axis.

Studies on the interaction between symptoms of panic and agoraphobia and family functioning are inconsistent. On the whole, marriages of people with panic disorder have not been found to be significantly different from those of couples without a member suffering from an anxiety disorder (28). Problems in these families may relate to difficulties dealing with a family member whose work and social functioning may be impaired and who may not be able to assume a full range of family responsibilities. Other problems are likely to be more specifically related to the particular issues in a given family. Family treatment in such situations, therefore, can only be effective if it follows a comprehensive assessment of the family.

Family members can also be enlisted as cotherapists in a patient's individual cognitive-behavioral treatment (29), and time can be allocated for spouses to share frustrations and concerns about the effect of symptoms on their relationship. Family members can help identify and correct the erroneous beliefs that may trigger panic symptoms. They can also support therapists' attempts at helping the patient realistically evaluate the probability that their worst fears will come to fruition. Most usefully, family members can be a significant help during behavioral components of therapy, when exposure to the feared objects and situations needs to be practiced to minimize the avoidance behavior, which ultimately reinforces the fear and anxiety. For family members to work together, they need to develop and reinforce effective communication and problem-solving skills. They need to negotiate an adjustment of role expectations while working on bringing symptoms of anxiety and avoidance under better control.

Expressed emotion, criticism, hostility, emotional overinvolvement, warmth, and positive regard in a family are related to treatment outcome with behavior therapy (30). Hostility and emotional overinvolvement are associated with more dropouts from treatment. Hostility by family members and a patient's perception of criticism are also significant predictors of poor outcome. As in other disorders, helping family members modulate the intensity of their interactions with each other both in terms of criticism or overinvolvement is helpful in dealing more effectively with psychiatric disorders within the family.

In general then, in addition to helping families deal with their particular concerns, the goals for family work with this population may most fruitfully focus on helping to cognitively reframe the experience and feared consequences of irrational perceptions and expectations, provide support to help individuals expose themselves to the feared stimulus, reduce levels of criticism and emotional overinvolvement, and help develop more effective communication and problem-solving skills.

Anxiety Disorders Case Example

Mrs. A, 36-year-old sales manager, presented with complaints of palpitations, anxiety, sweating, dizziness, and feeling faint. She could not identify a precipitant for her symptoms. She complained of feeling chronically uneasy and anxious. She had always been a shy, private, and sensitive person but had not needed professional care in the past to manage her situation. She came for help at this time because she was becoming afraid to go to work for fear of having an anxiety attack.

The intensity of her symptoms had been building for the past year and had gotten significantly worse over the previous 3 months. She denied feelings of depression. There was no change in her mood, appetite, energy, or concentration, but she did have difficulty falling asleep. Her family history was unremarkable except for the fact that her mother and aunt were also described as anxious.

Mrs. A was divorced at the age of 30, remarried 1 year later, and was living with her second husband and 16-year-old son from her first marriage. She liked her job. The work was stressful and demanding but a source of pride and satisfaction for her because it gave her a sense of competence and mastery. She was put on clonazepam 1 mg three times a day by her family doctor and found this gave significant relief. She wanted to continue the clonazepam despite discussions about the likelihood of tolerance and dependence.

After the initial evaluation, the psychiatrist asked to meet with Mrs. A together with her husband and son. She was initially reluctant to ask them to come as she felt that they would not be interested in participating in her treatment. When she did ask them to join her for a family meeting, she was surprised that they were willing.

At the first family meeting, the psychiatrist thanked them for coming and explained that he liked to see the families of all patients to try to understand their concerns, to give them a chance to ask questions, and to plan together the most appropriate next steps to take. He solicited their agreement to proceed with the evaluation. Next the psychiatrist asked each family member to outline problems that each person perceived.

Mr. A expressed concern about Mrs. A's symptoms, her nervousness, irritability, and distance from him. Mrs. A reiterated her concerns about her symptoms of anxiety and also brought up concerns about her son spending too much time away from home with friends. At first, her son was reluctant to discuss problems, but with support he identified a desire to spend more time with his biological father and his concern that Mr. A was trying to act too much like his father at home.

The therapist then proceeded to assess the family's functioning overall and along a number of domains outlined in the McMaster Model (see Chapter 4). Mr. and Mrs. A had trouble discussing emotionally sensitive issues, and the son felt uneasy talking about most things. The parents felt connected to each other emotionally, but Mr. A thought his wife was too close to her son, leaving him feeling left out. The son in turn felt she was most concerned about losing her husband at his expense. The family had worked out satisfactory allocation of roles and responsibilities except for the son, who tended to abdicate some of his responsibilities. The parents generally agreed on rules in the family and ways of dealing with transgressions, but Mr. A felt that Mrs. A was too ready to excuse her son, while she thought that he was too rigid and demanding.

Family intervention in anxiety disorders

- Enlist family members as cotherapists to help identify and correct erroneous beliefs, realistically evaluate probability of fears coming to fruition
- Help with practice to exposure to feared objects
- Reinforce effective communication and problem-solving skills
- Negotiate adjustment in role expectations
- Reduce emotional intensity of family interactions
- Reduce emotional overinvolvement

The psychiatrist shared his formulation with the family, suggesting that Mrs. A seemed to have a vulnerability to anxiety disorders, precipitated this time by the complexities of trying to maintain cohesiveness in the family at a time when her son was trying to become more independent by asserting his distance from her and by trying to connect more to his biological father. Mrs. A was afraid of losing her closeness with her son and tried to keep him close by being more accommodating. Mr. A was feeling threatened by the son's new assertiveness and by Mrs. A's attempts to appease her son. He reacted by trying to assert more control, leading to even greater conflict with both his wife and stepson. The psychiatrist gave the family an opportunity to share their thoughts about his formulation and to correct anything that did not fit their perception of their problems. The psychiatrist then asked the family members what, if anything, they wanted to do about changing the way they were dealing with their situation so as to make it less distressing for everybody.

The family members decided that they wanted to be able to talk about their anxieties more openly. Mrs. A felt that she needed more support from her husband to deal with her concerns about losing her son. Mr. A asked for more reassurance that his role in the family would continue to be important as the son moved to greater independence. He wanted the opportunity to spend more time with his wife in order to focus more on their relationship. The son wanted to feel free to be able to spend more time with his biological father without being made to feel guilty.

Over the next four meetings, the therapist met with the family to follow up on how they were able to change their interactions. They decided to have dinner together as a family at least three times a week, during which time they would discuss more openly how they were doing and how they would deal with new concerns. The son agreed that he would see more of his father, but only after he completed the chores that were part of his responsibilities in the home. The parents went out at least once a week together to a movie or a walk or restaurant to allow time to focus on their relationship. At the same time the husband and son were encouraged to help Mrs. A face her anxiety by supporting her to continue to go out and participate in the world despite fears that she might develop an anxiety attack. They learned it was most helpful for her to practice facing her fears to become desensitized to them.

The psychiatrist weaned Mrs. A off the clonazepam and started her on sertraline, which she tolerated well. With the antidepressant, exposure therapy, and family work, Mrs. A's symptoms diminished significantly and she was able to continue to work effectively.

Obsessive-Compulsive Disorder

Obsessive-compulsive disorder is thought to originate from some form of neurodevelopmental abnormality. There is no evidence that any particular types of family interactional processes play a role in the etiology of the disorder (31). As with other disorders, the way a family deals with symptoms can influence the evolution of the disorder.

Patients with obsessive-compulsive disorder are more likely to be single than those with other forms of anxiety disorders. Many of these patients live with their families of origin, who are often caught up in the ritualistic behavior of their loved ones. Many families of patients with obsessive-compulsive disorder report having distressed relationships (32, 33), although their average scores on most marital satisfaction measures are unremarkable.

High expressed emotion in families has also been found to be predictive of relapse for patients with obsessive-compulsive disorder (34, 35). Hostile criticism is particularly problematic, as is excessive accommodation to the patient's rituals (36).

The mainstay of psychosocial treatment for obsessive-compulsive disorder involves exposure and response prevention strategies in a behavioral therapy format, usually provided in conjunction with pharmacotherapy aimed at reducing the intensity of the obsessive and compulsive symptoms and treating comorbid conditions (e.g., major depression). As with panic disorder, family involvement in the treatment of patients with obsessive-compulsive disorder usually consists of assisting family members' support of a behavioral therapy program. This can be done with individual families or in a multifamily group format (37). Family involvement in the treatment of obsessive-compulsive disorders does not appear to lead to a significant reduction of symptoms but has been found helpful in improving family relationships and in decreasing the likelihood of relapse (38).

Specific aspects of helpful approaches with families of patients with obsessive-compulsive disorders include educating families about the illness and available treatments and helping families to reduce accommodation to the obsessive-compulsive rituals (39). Family work is particularly helpful in children with obsessive-compulsive disorder. Studies have focused on providing psychoeducation, distancing from the child's symptoms, reducing family conflict and disruptions, supporting relaxation training for the child, parental anxiety management, and problem-solving skills training (40, 41).

Family functioning in patients with obsessive-compulsive disorders depends on many variables, including severity of the patient's symptoms, responsiveness to treatment, patient and families' coping skills and support systems, their understanding of the illness, and the degree to which symptoms are contained by the patient or are disruptive to the functioning of other family members. For those patients whose symptoms are poorly controlled, patients who spend extensive periods of time participating in their rituals, and patients whose rituals affect the daily lives of their family members, family dysfunction is to be expected, and including family members in treatment is particularly important. Determination of which family member needs treatment and the degree of involvement of family members in the treatment should be individualized. During the family assessment, it is evident what the needs of the family are and to what extent they can be an aid or hindrance to the patient's treatment. In this perspective, treatment for families of patients with obsessive-compulsive disorder is no different than for any other illness.

Research findings can inform a therapist's approach to a family with obsessive-compulsive disorder. Helping family members reduce excess criticism or overinvolvement may help to delay relapse once symptom reduction has been achieved. An important part of the family meetings is the provision of information and education about the illness. Family members can learn to not blame each other and to appreciate the distress patients may be experiencing from their symptoms. They can be enlisted to help with exposure and response prevention exercises the patient needs to practice. In addition, family members can be helped to decrease their accommodation to the patient's rituals and to communicate and problem solve more effectively.

Obsessive-Compulsive Disorder Case Example

David was a 17-year-old male who presented with complaints of long-standing symptoms of compulsive behaviors that were becoming increasingly out of control. He was having trouble functioning in school and was creating major disturbances at home. He was preoccupied with germs and cleanliness. He was afraid to touch surfaces with his hands and used tissues whenever he needed to touch objects, leaving tissues around the house after using them. He spent inordinate amounts of time cleaning himself in the bathroom but inevitably left the space in much greater disarray than when he started, creating major problems for the rest of his family. David felt very badly about himself, isolated himself from his peers by staying at home, and ate constantly in an attempt to soothe himself. He became morbidly obese.

David's older brother did not have psychiatric problems and was successfully attending university out of town. His mother and father were in constant conflict over differences in how they dealt with David's symptoms. His mother alternated between appeasing him because she felt sorry for him and becoming angry at the disruptions he was creating in the home. She was distressed enough herself to require psychiatric care for depression and anxiety. His father had given up in frustration at not being able to have any impact on these behaviors and had withdrawn from attempting to help in any meaningful way.

David was diagnosed with obsessive-compulsive disorder by a psychiatrist who put him on fluvoxamine and referred him to a psychotherapist for a program of exposure and response prevention relating to his fear of dirt. In addition, the psychiatrist met with David and his parents to try to better understand the social context in which David's pharmacotherapy and psychological treatment were to take place.

Family intervention in OCD

- Reduce criticism and emotional overinvolvement
- Provide information and education about the illness and treatments available
- Reduce blame, appreciate distress
- Help with exposure and response prevention
- Decrease accommodations to rituals
- Improve communication and problem solving

In the first meeting the psychiatrist welcomed David and his parents to the family meeting. He explained that he likes to meet with the families of all of his patients to get a better understanding of how everybody sees the problems, to provide the opportunity to ask questions, and to plan together how to proceed. Once the family agreed to the purpose of the meeting, he asked them to describe how they saw the problems in the family.

The mother was very frustrated by David's disruptive behaviors and the consequences they were having, both for David's ability to function in school and socially and for the chaos he created at home. She was also upset about her husband's lack of involvement in finding better solutions to David's illness. The father was similarly frustrated by David's symptoms and their impact on their lives. He was critical of his wife's inconsistent response to his son's symptomatic behavior, which alternated between trying to accommodate and trying to set limits for him. David felt very badly about his preoccupation with contamination and inability to control his behaviors. He missed being able to socialize with others his own age. He felt estranged from his father, feeling that his father was very critical and did not like him. He was also upset about the bickering and tension that he sensed between his parents.

The psychiatrist then reviewed the family's functioning along a variety of other domains as outlined in the McMaster Model. He noted that all family members had difficulties in communicating, particularly around emotional issues. They had difficulty coming to a consensus about how to resolve problems. David felt emotionally connected with his mother, whom he saw as very concerned about his welfare, but he felt that his father was disengaged from him. Both the mother and the father felt that they were increasingly in their own worlds and not supportive of each other in dealing with this chronic illness and unremitting symptoms. Family roles and responsibilities were satisfactorily assigned and carried out except by David, who because of his rituals had a great deal of difficulty in completing anything in a timely manner. The parents also disagreed about rules and ways of dealing with limits and expectations in the family.

The psychiatrist formulated for the family that in his view David's obsessive-compulsive disorder was likely based on biological vulnerability that was not his or his family's fault. David's illness had created a significant burden for the family, a burden that the family was having difficulty dealing with. The family had difficulty discussing the emotional impact of the illness and supporting each other. Their different ways of dealing with the problem without coming to a mutually agreed approach made a difficult situation even more difficult. Once the family agreed with the formulation, the psychiatrist asked them to outline ways in which they thought they would like to see improvement, not only in David's illness but also in their ways of dealing with it. The family wanted to focus on becoming more comfortable talking with each other in a noncritical and supportive manner. The parents wanted to have the opportunity to spend some time together without focusing on David's problems. David wanted to be able to do things with his father to begin to reestablish a connection that was more positive.

Over six family sessions, the psychiatrist helped the family implement those goals by having them follow through on the commitments that they had made to each other. He helped them stay on track and continue to make the necessary effort to bring about the changes they all wanted. If they were successful in following through on their assigned tasks, he was supportive of those efforts. If they had difficulty in keeping to their assignments, he reviewed with them why and helped them to adjust their efforts or their goals so as to improve the likelihood that they could be successful. He also provided them more education and information about obsessive-compulsive disorders. He helped them to be less critical with each other and helped David's mother become less focused on him. He also supported them to persist in complying with medications and the exposure and response prevention–based psychotherapy. There was some improvement in David's obsessive behaviors over time, but the illness continued as an ongoing problem. The family became more adept at helping David to manage his illness more effectively. Over time, the impact of the illness became much less disturbing both for David and for his family.

Conclusion

Psychiatric illness affects the functioning of families. Family functioning, in turn, influences the course and outcome of the psychiatric illness. Different disorders present some common challenges to the families of patients. Each family, however, deals with these challenges in its own unique ways depending on the composition of the family, age of family members, their socioeconomic status, family developmental stage, available resources, presence or absence of other family stresses, and health of other family members. To provide optimal treatment, therapists need to become familiar with the effect of illnesses on patients and their significant others and also to assess how the patients' social support system is functioning so that any help required can be targeted to their specific needs. Although information is available in the literature, much research still needs to be undertaken to guide therapists in accomplishing both of these goals.

References

1. Addington S, Collins A, Addington D: The role of family work in early psychosis. Schizophr Res 79:77–83, 2005
2. McFarlane WR, Dixon L, Lukens E, et al: Family psychoeducation and schizophrenia: a review of the literature. J Marital Fam Ther 29:223–245, 2003
3. American Psychiatric Association Work Group on Schizophrenia: Practice guideline for the treatment of patients with schizophrenia, 2nd edition. Am J Psychiatry 161 (2 suppl):1–56, 2004
4. Dyck DG, Hendryx MS, Short RA, et al: Service use among patients with schizophrenia in psychoeducational multiple-family group treatment. Psychiatr Serv 53:749–754, 2002
5. Chien WT, Chan SW: One-year follow-up of a multiple-family group intervention for Chinese families of patients with schizophrenia. Psychiatr Serv 55:1276–1284, 2004

6. Rummel CB, Hansen WP, Helbig A, et al: Peer-to-peer psychoeducation in schizophrenia: a new approach. J Clin Psychiatry 66:1580–1585, 2005

7. Dixon L, Lucksted A, Stewart B, et al: Outcomes of the peer-taught 12-week family-to-family education program for severe mental illness. Acta Psychiatr Scand 109:207–215, 2004

8. Tsuchiya KJ, Byrne M, Morteuseu PB: Risk factors in relation to an emergence of bipolar disorder: a systematic review. Bipolar Disord 5:231–242, 2003

9. Hooley JM, Woodberry KA, Ferriter C: Family factors in schizophrenia and bipolar disorder, in Psychotherapy and the Family. Edited by Hudson JL, Rapee RM. Amsterdam, Elsevier, 2005, pp 205–223

10. Keitner GI, Ryan CE, Heur A: Families of people with bipolar disorder, in Families and Mental Disorders: From Burden to Empowerment. Edited by Sartorius N, Leff J, Lopez-Ibor J, et al. Hoboken, NJ, Wiley, 2005, pp 69–85

11. Dore G, Romans SE: Impact of bipolar affective disorder on family and partners. J Affect Disord 67:147–158, 2001

12. Walsh F: Clinical views of family normality, health, and dysfunction, in Normal Family Process. Edited by Walsh F. New York, Guilford, 2003, pp 27–57

13. Keitner GI, Solomon DA, Ryan CE, et al: Prodromal and residual symptoms in bipolar 1 disorder. Compr Psychiatry 37:362–367, 1996

14. Keitner GI, Miller IW: Family functioning and major depression: an overview. Am J Psychiatry 147:1128–1137, 1990

15. Gaber J: Depression and the family, in Psychotherapy and the Family. Edited by Hudson JJ, Ropee RM. Amsterdam, Elsevier, 2005, pp 225–280

16. Gupta M, Beach SRH, Coyne JC: Optimizing couple and parenting interventions to address adult depression, in Handbook of Clinical Family Therapy. Edited by Lebow JL. Hoboken, NJ, Wiley, 2005, pp 228–250

17. Butzlaff RI, Hooley JM: Expressed emotion and psychiatric relapse. Arch Gen Psychiatry 55:547–552, 1998

18. Keitner GI, Ryan CE, Miller IW, et al: Psychosocial factors and the long term course of major depression. J Affect Disord 44:57–67, 1997

19. Leff J, Vearnals S, Brewin CR: The London Depression Intervention Trial: randomized controlled trial of antidepressants v. couple therapy in the treatment and maintenance of people with depression living with a partner; clinical outcome and costs. Br J Psychiatry 177:95–100, 2000

20. O'Farrell TJ, Fals-Stewart W: Behavioral couples therapy for alcoholism and drug abuse. J Subst Abuse Treat 18:51–54, 2000

21. Fals-Stewart W, Klostermann K, Yates BT, et al: Brief relationship therapy for alcoholism: a randomized clinical trial examining clinical efficacy and cost-effectiveness. Psychol Addict Behav 19:363–371, 2005

22. Fals-Stewart W, Birchler GR: A national survey of the use of couples therapy in substance abuse treatment. J Subst Abuse Treat 20:277–283, 2001

23. Steketee G, Fogler J: Families of people with a severe anxiety disorder, in Families and Mental Disorders: From Burden to Empowerment. Edited by Sartorius N, Leff J, Lopez-Ibor J, et al. Hoboken, NJ, Wiley, pp 87–112, 2005

24. Barlow DH: Anxiety and Its Disorders: The Nature and Treatment of Anxiety and Panic, 2nd Edition. New York, Guilford Press, 2002

25. Goldstein AJ, Chambless DL: Reanalysis of agoraphobia. Behav Ther 9:47–59, 1978

26. Ballenger JC: Toward an integrated model of panic disorder. Am J Orthopsychiatry 59:284–293, 1989

27. Kahn RS, Asnis GM, Wetzler S, et al: Neuroendocrine evidence for serotonin hypersensitivity in panic disorder. Psychopharmacology 96:360–364, 1988

28. Carter MM, Tuvorsky J, Barlow DH: Interpersonal relationships in panic disorder with agoraphobia: a review of empirical evidence. Clin Psychol Sci Pract 1:25–34, 1994

29. Gore KL, Carter MM: Family therapy for panic disorder: a cognitive-behavioral interpersonal approach to treatment, in Family Therapy and Mental Health: Innovations in Therapy and Practice. Edited by MacFarlane MM. New York, Haworth, 2001, pp 109–134

30. Chambless DL, Steketee G: Expressed emotion and behavior therapy outcome: a positive study with obsessive-compulsive and agoraphobic outpatients. J Consult Clin Psychol 67:658–665, 1999

31. Steketee G, Pruyn N: Family functioning in OCD, in Obsessive Compulsive Disorder: Theory, Research, and Treatment. Edited by Swinson RP, Antony MM, Rachman S, et al. New York, Guilford, 1998, pp 120–140

32. Steketee G: Disability and family burden in obsessive-compulsive disorder. Can J Psychiatry 42:919–928, 1997

33. Emmelkamp PMG, de Haan E, Hoogdvin CAL: Marital adjustment and obsessive-compulsive disorder. Br J Psychiatry 156:55–60, 1990

34. Emmelkamp PMG, Van Dyck R, Bitter M, et al: Spouse-aided therapy with agoraphobics. Br J Psychiatry 160:51–56, 1992

35. Chambless DL, Bryan AD, Aiken LS, et al: Predicting expressed emotion: a study with families of obsessive-compulsive and agoraphobic outpatients. J Fam Psychol 15:225–240, 2001

36. Amir N, Freshman M, Foa EB: Family distress and involvement in relatives of obsessive-compulsive disorder patients. J Anxiety Disord 14:209–217, 2000

37. Van Noppen B, Steketee G, McCorkle BH, et al: Group and multifamily behavioral treatment for obsessive-compulsive disorder: a pilot study. J Anxiety Disord 11:431–446, 1997

38. MacFarlane MM: Systemic treatment of obsessive-compulsive disorders in a rural community mental health center: an integrative approach, in Family Therapy and Mental Health: Innovations in Therapy and Practice. Edited by MacFarlane MM. Binghamton, NY, Haworth Clinical Practice Press, 2001, pp 155–183

39. Grunes MS, Neziroglu F, McKay D: Family involvement in the behavioral treatment of obsessive-compulsive disorder: a preliminary investigation. Behav Ther 32:803–820, 2001

40. Piacentini J, Bergman RL, Jacobs C, et al: Open trial of cognitive behavior therapy for childhood obsessive compulsive disorder. J Anxiety Disord 16:207–219, 2002

41. Waters TL, Barrett PM, March JS: Cognitive-behavioral family treatment of childhood obsessive-compulsive disorder: preliminary findings. Am J Psychother 55:372–387, 2001

12

Special Situations

- Apply general principles of assessment and treatment to all combinations of people who consider themselves a family.
- Be sensitive to and understand the role of gender, race, culture, and sexual orientation.
- Understand laws in your state with respect to reporting child/elder abuse.
- Follow specific steps required for assessment and treatment of intimate partner violence.

The general principles of assessment and treatment can be applied to all combinations and constellations of people who consider themselves a family even as the content of the specific presenting situation may change. The basic approach should be similar: connect with the family, assess and identify the problems, develop a formulation, outline options for the family to choose, and help them to actualize their goals. However, some situations can benefit from reference to a specific and unique body of knowledge and to the acquisition of additional specific skills. This chapter is not intended to be inclusive but provides direction about certain specific clinical situations.

Therapeutic Alliance: Gender, Race, Culture, and Sexual Orientation

A good therapeutic alliance is a predictor of good outcome in couples therapy. The therapeutic alliance is influenced by many factors, from individual psychopathology to the physical differences between patient and therapist. Individuals with early family distress and subsequent attachment disorders or personality disorders are more likely to have difficulty forming positive alliances in couples therapy (1). Age can be a powerful factor, with younger therapists being reluctant to address issues of sexuality with couples who may be the age of their parents. Older female therapists are frequently cast as a mother figure, with either positive or negative connotations.

The immediate perceptions of therapists and couples remain well established into mid-treatment. The strength of a woman's alliance is especially predictive of good outcome (2). However, when men's alliances were stronger at session eight, couples showed most improvement. The racial background of the couples was not statistically significant for the formation of the initial alliance, although early terminators contained more African Americans and fewer Caucasians. Clinicians have suggested that working harder to engage the male partner at the beginning of therapy may help the therapist establish the most positive therapeutic alliance with the couple. It may also be worthwhile to work harder to ensure a good alliance when ethnic or racial difference is present.

It is common for a partner of the same sex as the therapist to solicit "gender solidarity" in an argument with his or her spouse. Triangulation can also occur with the opposite-sex partner trying to seek a seductive connection with the therapist. The therapist must avoid taking sides and being drawn into a split (3). Therapists can reduce perceived bias by seeking agreement at each stage of the assessment, following up where a family member seems hesitant or unsure, and making certain that the concerns and needs of all family members are addressed.

Family roles are still highly stratified by gender, with women performing most of the emotional caregiving in the family even when both partners work full time. Role allocation and division of labor can be problematic. Although male partners are increasingly taking on day-to-day responsibilities in managing a household, it is usually at the direction of the female partner. Expectations about what is important, how problems are best addressed (practically or emotionally), and how to combine the pressures of work, parenting, and home maintenance create areas of potential conflict. The therapist needs to be able to view problems as based in cultural norms as well as personal pathology or family dysfunction.

Culture and Race

It is important to develop a strong working alliance when ethnic or racial differences are present. Patients may hide their reactions from the psychiatrist out of culturally sanctioned beliefs such as fear of rejection if there is a disagreement or through deference to authority. Patients and families may also get angry if they feel slighted or misunderstood. Well-meaning therapists may hold egalitarian beliefs but may not be aware of subtle negative attitudes and stereotypes about people of color or may not have had sufficient contact with people different from themselves. Strategies to reduce bias and to promote a healthy and constructive therapeutic alliance include increasing awareness of possible negative attitudes, immersing oneself in other cultural experiences, working hard to stay attuned to patients, demonstrating cultural empathy, and being respectful and open to alternative worldviews (4).

Historical racism may interfere with an African American patient's seeking treatment (5). Ethnic minority populations underutilize psychotherapy services and have high rates of dropping out of treatment (6). Dovidio et al. (7) demonstrated in a series of studies that contemporary racism among Caucasians is subtle, often unintentional, and unconscious. White physicians may display negative body language (less eye contact, voice tone not as warm or natural) in response to those who are different from themselves. Caucasians who demonstrate these behaviors report not being aware of this negativity. Members of ethnic minority groups, however, were aware of negative attitudes toward them in studies that examined these interactions. A genogram can be used to explore how the family understands culture difference and ethnicity and can also be used as a training tool for therapists (8).

It is always important to recognize that "cultural" issues can sometimes be best understood as family problems that need to be resolved. For example, Mrs. J, who is Catholic, and Mr. J, who is Jewish, fought about how to celebrate the December holidays. Exploration revealed that neither member of the couple had been very religious before marriage and had seldom celebrated holidays. However, when Mrs. J's father died and her mother became depressed, Mrs. J began to spend more time with her mother, a very religious woman, and was less available to her husband. Conflict over her return to her family of origin was being expressed by the couple through their inability to compromise over religious rituals (9).

Cultural competence means being aware of one's own attitudes, being knowledgeable about cultural issues, and having the clinical skills to understand the cultural context of the patient's concerns. Establishing rapport with a patient can be enhanced by listening to the patient's story. Demonstrating humility and concern can also be effective in this regard, although the former is not a common physician characteristic. Self-reflection regarding personal, institutional, internalized, and subtle forms of bias is an important part of cultural competence in general. Cultural competence training requires both general attitudinal approaches and specific advice based on cultural aspects of minority life. Some teachers, concerned about stereotyping, discourage the knowledge approach to cultural competence training and argue that cultural humility is superior to cultural competence. Cultural competence education should be tailored for the ethnic and racial minorities that are present in the community served by specific health care providers. However, when faced with an unfamiliar culture, the therapist can ask the family members to talk about their culture and what important information the therapist should know in order to be of help. This position of naïveté helps engage the family and encourages a sense of competence in the family (10).

Although the Problem-Centered Systems Therapy of the Family (PCSTF) was developed in a Judeo-Christian cultural context, it can be used easily in different cultural contexts. The PCSTF is focused on the identified problems and needs of each family with the goal of reaching a consensus about the family's concerns and intentions toward change. The therapist may have opinions about the presenting problems and may share them with the family, but unless there is a safety issue, it is up to the family what the goals of treatment should be. These goals may well be different in families from different cultural backgrounds. It is the role of the therapist to help the family resolve problems in a way that is compatible with the family's belief systems and cultural norms.

Sexual Minorities

Sexual minority patients rate female clinicians as more helpful than heterosexual male clinicians (11). In this study, 392 lesbian and gay clients described the most important therapeutic practices as those that convey sensitivity to and awareness and appreciation of sexual minority status. Nine negative practices were identified, including "your therapist indicated that he or she believed that a gay or lesbian identity is bad, sick, or inferior," "your therapist pressured or advised you to come out to someone in spite of the fact that you believed it was too risky," and "your therapist apparently did not understand the problems of societal prejudice against gay men and lesbians and/or internalized homophobia." Four supportive practices were also identified, including "your therapist never made an issue of your sexual orientation when it was not relevant" and "your therapist helped you feel good about yourself as a gay man or lesbian." This finding is consistent with the findings of other clinicians and researchers who have suggested it is important for clinicians to provide a gay-affirming environment for sexual minorities (12). More empirical investigations are needed to identify specific therapeutic interventions that contribute to good outcome for same-sex couples (13). As with culture, the PCSTF applies to same-sex couples as it does to heterosexual couples. The assessment should focus on areas of functioning that are problematic or that work well, with the goal of helping to change the former and reinforce the latter. Issues of communications, problem solving, role allocation, emotional connectedness, and safe behavior are common to all families even if details of what family functions should be vary with a given couple.

Competing Value Systems

Physicians often find it hard not to impose their own values: "Surely it is wrong for a woman to be beaten? She must leave her husband!" "Abortion is wrong." "Multiple sex partners should not be condoned." When does the therapist "help" the woman leave an abusive marriage? When does the therapist "help" the adolescent girl leave a family who is forcing her to marry a man she doesn't love? When can therapists say that they do not want to work with a family because they disagree with the family's values?

If competing value systems cannot be resolved, the therapist may need to either refer the couple or family elsewhere or get supervision. In either case, the therapist should say up front to the family that there are competing value systems that may preclude a good working relationship. This should be discussed at length and a solution agreed upon. In most cases the disagreement can be framed as a different way of looking at things, but in cases that involve common social beliefs about neglect or mistreatment, the psychiatrist should be clear about the nature of the inability to treat the family. For example, the therapist may hold specific traditional views about marriage and may find it difficult to treat couples with "open marriages." Usually, however, the problem is the inverse, with the therapist holding more liberal views and the couple or family holding more traditional views. The traditional deferential role of women, for example, can be particularly hard for female physicians to grapple with, and it may also be hard for a traditional patriarchal family to accept the female physician as a valid authority figure.

The role of the therapist, in our view, is to provide a safe environment in which families can discuss their concerns and negotiate mutually agreed-upon alternatives. The therapist should not enforce his or her own values but instead meet the family where they are most comfortable so that whatever solutions are developed will be more likely to persist.

Affairs

Affairs occur relatively frequently in relationships, can be devastating, and are a common presenting problem in couples therapy. Affairs are one of the most complicated issues to assess and treat. Despite this, there are very few empirical studies on family treatment of infidelity.

The general family therapy literature on affairs presumes the cultural norm of long-term monogamous partnerships as ideal and healthy. It does not account for individuals, cultures, and subcultures that consider monogamy a relative value. In the gay community, it is not uncommon for couples to choose nonmonogamous sexual arrangements with the commitment in the primary relationship being mostly about emotional fidelity, attachment, and dependability rather than sexual faithfulness (14). The decision to have an affair and the meaning of an affair relate to an individual's implicit or explicit sociocultural construction of marriage or committed relationships.

People seek out an affair for many reasons, including sexual gratification, emotional connection, self-discovery, novelty, freedom, or a wish to recapture lost parts of the self, recapture vitality, or counteract feelings of disappointment, emptiness, or constraint. Affairs can also be the result of individual psychopathology such as attachment disorders. Affairs can be about fantasy and illusions or anger and revenge. Sometimes the reason is related to feeling vulnerable in a particular moment of the life cycle, such as the birth of a child, the loss of a parent, or being "empty nested." Affairs may arise from confusion regarding one's sexual orientation, sexual addictions, and acts of retaliation. The motivations for having an affair also vary according to gender. For men, an affair may be motivated by a sense of entitlement, such as the middle-aged man who, feeling prosperous, leaves his aging wife for a younger partner, or the philanderer whose self-esteem is based on his number of conquests. For women, motivation may be related to romantic ideals, disappointments with their bargain in the marriage, or rebelliousness related to a sense of constriction associated with the burdens of domesticity.

A segmented model of marriage is common in some European and Latin American cultures. In this arrangement, the two partners enter the relationship with the expectation that the marriage will fulfill some needs but not others. Autonomy is highly valued, marriage and affairs are seen as separate domains, and affairs are presumed to be a private matter. The first step in assessing a couple in which there is acknowledged infidelity is to understand what assumptions and expectations each partner brings to the marriage. If the couple enters treatment, their assumptions will influence the expectations and needs in treatment.

Case Example

A couple presents for an assessment with the complaint, not that the husband was having an affair, but that he brought his girlfriend home when his wife was out of town. The therapist asks, "How was it agreed that it was okay for Don to have affairs?" Don replied that Susan herself was having a lesbian affair and that they both tolerated each other's sexual behavior outside of the relationship. They said they had an open marriage. Susan replied, "Everything was fine and dandy until you decided to bring Jane home when I was away on business. I don't mind you having these flings but what I really mind is you bringing her home and humiliating me in front of our friends." During the assessment, the couple acknowledged each other's point of view and spontaneously agreed to make changes according to the other's wishes. Susan said, in summary, at the end of the assessment, "I just wanted him to hear me out in a public setting. I am satisfied he has heard me and will not have Jane over again." While the therapist may have identified other problems within the relationship, the couple did not recognize a need to correct other aspects of their relationship. The therapist's belief about marriage is less relevant than the couple's. What is important is to assess the couple's agreement or disagreement on the problems and what they want to do about the problems.

Couples dealing with an affair

Stage 1
- Impact of affair; stabilization and affect containment
- Assessment of current functioning
- Development of shared treatment plan

Stage 2
- Effect of the affair
- Improved communication
- Provision of explanation for affair

Stage 3
- Recovery and moving on
- Forgiveness

Most couples come to treatment to deal with the impact of an affair. The impact varies according to whether the affair is disclosed or unintentionally discovered. It is important to recognize that women are more harshly punished if discovered. Men are less forgiving and more prone to revenge and acts of violence; in the United States, men divorce their wives for infidelity more often than wives divorce their husbands (15). Transparency and truth-telling are highly valued in the United States, whereas in other cultures, such as those in Africa, the Middle East, Latin America, and Europe, avoiding confrontation, keeping information private, and lying are seen as protective of the partner and the relationship. The belief in the family therapy field in the United States has been that intimacy emerges from working through the trauma of disclosure. This belief is now being challenged by therapists such as Scheinkman (16), who offers an alternative approach advocating acknowledgment of each partner's perspective and the provision of a holding environment for the couple as key treatment elements. The therapist's attitude is essential in lending hope to the couple that they will be able to "get to the other side" and in creating a constructive and safe process for reflection and decision making.

Evidence suggests that couples who had an affair and who revealed this affair prior to or during therapy show greater improvement in satisfaction than couples who had not had affairs. The couples who had affairs improve in therapy at a greater rate, particularly at the end of therapy, and the outcome of couples who had an affair can be indistinguishable from the outcome of distressed couples without affairs (17). It should be noted that treatments that address the whole relationship are likely to be more successful than treatments that focus on the affair (18).

One model that has been tested empirically and found effective in couples dealing with an affair describes three stages (18). Stage 1 deals with the impact of the affair on each individual. It is important when assessing current functioning to identify relationship strengths and develop a shared treatment plan. The couple will need to negotiate boundaries; amount of time spent with each other or apart; whether to continue their sexual relationship; if, when, and how to terminate contact with the outside person; and what information to share with others, if any. Attention also needs to be paid to appropriate self-care, such as continued social contact with others, some degree of disengagement, and what constitutes appropriate venting with others. This initial phase is focused on stabilization and affective containment.

Stage 2 allows for the examination of the effect of the affair on the relationship and on the individuals themselves. Effective communication must be accompanied by affective regulation in spite of the hurt that may be experienced by the injured party. This stage has the goal of providing an explanation for the affair and sets the groundwork for the third stage, which is focused on recovery and moving on. Stage 3 also works on forgiveness, including being released from the control of negative affect toward the partner.

Violence

Family violence can consist of physical, verbal, or sexual abuse against a partner, child, or elder. Physical violence is an act that directly threatens a family member's safety. Verbal or emotional abuse involves a symbolic threat, such as threats of abandonment or injury, derogatory comments, and insults. Sexual abuse involves acts that are coercive, sexually aggressive, or exploitative. A combination of these forms of violence is often present in families where violence is prevalent.

The term *domestic violence* emerged in the United States with the rise of the women's movement in the 1970s. Prior to this, violence between partners was considered a private matter. A specific type of domestic violence, known as *intimate partner violence* (IPV), refers to violence between marital partners. We are most aware of the type of IPV in which one partner is the aggressor and the other partner is the victim. Public awareness campaigns and educational programs have encouraged victims of domestic violence to seek help through hotlines and have provided safe houses or shelters for women and children fleeing violent spouses. Twenty-five percent of U.S. women report being victims of partner violence during their lifetime, and 1.5 million women and 835,000 men report physical or sexual assault annually (19). It may be surprising to note the high prevalence of male victims.

The first step in the treatment of violence consists of a comprehensive assessment of individual functioning. Individual psychopathology such as organic mental conditions, delusional disorders, paranoid schizophrenia, substance abuse, and personality disorders may be contributing and should be treated appropriately. It may not be possible to conduct family therapy until the individual pathology is stabilized. Family members have to be able to agree to abstain from violence during the course of therapy in order for the therapy to be successful. If an individual is unable to control violent urges, even for a limited time, a more restrictive level of care is needed, either hospitalization or incarceration.

The mandatory and optional reporting laws for violence vary from state to state, and each psychiatrist must be knowledgeable about particular state laws. It is also important to inform patients of the limitations of confidentiality prior to beginning therapy. In the case of child or elder abuse, making a report of family violence can be empowering by helping the perpetrating family members begin to take control of their impulses and the victims to feel protected. Dangerous weapons should be removed from the home. It is only when safety is assured that the necessary steps can begin to be taken to understand the precipitants and antecedents to the violence and alternative ways of dealing with difficulties developed. Countertransference problems can be problematic in working with families with violence and abuse. The therapist needs to be able to form an alliance with both victim and perpetrator. Psychiatrists should seek consultation and perhaps work with a cotherapist, if necessary, when families present with these particularly challenging problems.

Exclusion factors for couples therapy

- Uncontrolled continuous use of alcohol or substances
- Fear of serious injury from partner
- Severe violence that has resulted in the recipient requiring medical attention
- Conviction for a violent crime or violation of a restraining order
- Prior use of a weapon against the partner
- Prior threat to kill the partner
- Stalking or other partner-focused obsessional behavior

Reciprocal physical violence is more common than generally known. In the U.S. National Comorbidity Survey (20), 6.5% of females and 5.5% of males reported reciprocal physical violence. In the 2001 National Longitudinal Study of Adolescent Health, which assessed subjects ages 18–28 years (21), violence was reported in 24% of all relationships, with 49% of relationships showing reciprocal violence. In cases of nonreciprocal violence, women were the perpetrators in 70% of cases. Reciprocity was associated with more frequent violence among women but not men. However, men were more likely to inflict injury than women, and reciprocal violence was associated with more injury than nonreciprocal violence, regardless of the gender of the perpetrator. The fact that women are frequent aggressors has also been identified in a meta-analysis of 82 studies (22). In fact, women are slightly more likely than men to report using physical aggression in intimate relationships, according to Archer (22). These findings are also reported in couples seeking outpatient treatment, in which 61% of husbands and 64% of wives were classified as aggressive (23). In a sample of inpatients hospitalized with suicidality, over 90% reported severe physical violence (24). Male and female patients in this study did not differ significantly on violence perpetration or victimization.

With reciprocal violence, serious injury generally does not occur, and the couple may not consider the violence a major relational problem. It seems most likely that there is a spectrum of IPV, with patriarchal male-to-female aggression being the most commonly recognized and the most serious in terms of physical and psychological injury to the female. However, a lesser form of IPV, with reciprocal IPV, may be more common.

What should the general psychiatrist know about screening for IPV and about treatment referral? What questions should be asked, and should the psychiatrist look for reciprocity? If couples request couples therapy, what should the psychiatrist advise? Good clinical practice includes asking questions about violence in the routine assessment. There are a number of places where these questions can seamlessly be included. It is important to provide a context in which to ask about violence. Under Affective Responsiveness, when asking about anger, the following questions can be asked: "Often when people are angry they throw things, push the other person, and yell a lot. Does that happen with you?" If the answer is yes, these follow-up questions can be asked: "Do you each play an equal part? Who usually starts it? Can you tell me how it usually happens?" It is vital to be able to differentiate serious violence that puts someone in the family at risk of injury versus the more common and less severe reciprocal "push and shove" violence. Questions should also assess the severity of injury sustained by the victim (e.g., What is the worst you have ever been injured by your partner? Have you ever sought medical attention from an injury sustained from your partner?). If the question seems relevant, the couple should be asked about the presence of guns in the home. Additionally, the clinician should be aware that the victim of violence might be unable to acknowledge the violence in the presence of the perpetrator. If the clinician suspects this is the case, he or she should conduct individual interviews to assess for violence. If violence is revealed in the individual interview, the clinician should provide safety planning.

What about couples who request help with IPV? When should couples therapy be recommended? The essential components of safe couples treatment include adequate screening out of couples where there is risk for severe IPV (25). The aim for the general psychiatrist is to exclude severe violence and recommend separate treatment for the victims and perpetrators. The following factors can be used to screen out severe IPV couples: uncontrolled continuous use of alcohol or substances, fear of serious injury from the partner, severe violence that has resulted in the recipient requiring medical attention, conviction for a violent crime or violation of a restraining order, prior use of a weapon against the partner, prior threat to kill the partner, stalking or other partner-focused obsessional behavior, and any bizarre forms of violence such as sadistic violence. If any of these factors are present, couples treatment is not recommended. If severe IPV is present, safety planning must be discussed with the individual at risk. This should include education about how to maintain safety, including the safety of dependents, and specifically how to access services in the community, including obtaining a restraining order.

Safety planning

- Memorize important phone numbers of people to call in emergency
- If your children are old enough, teach them important phone numbers, including when to dial 911
- Keep information about domestic violence in a safe place, where your abuser won't find it but you can get it when you need to review it
- Always have change for pay phones and/or access to a mobile phone
- If you can, open your own bank account
- Stay in touch with friends
- Get to know your neighbors
- Don't cut yourself off from other people, even if you feel you want to be alone
- Rehearse your escape plan until you know it by heart
- Leave with a trusted friend or relative the following: a set of car keys, extra money, a change of clothes, and copies of important documents, including your own and your children's birth certificates, children's school and medical records, bank books, welfare identification, passport/green card, immigration papers, Social Security card, lease agreements or mortgage payment books, insurance papers, important addresses and telephone numbers

---

For couples with reciprocal violence who wish to enter couples therapy, it is still important to ensure safety. The key components to safe couples therapy include the signing of a no-violence contract, the use of a negotiated time-out tool, and strategies to manage anger. Treatment of comorbidity is also important, and in addition to alcohol screening, patients and their partners should be assessed for depressive disorders and posttraumatic stress disorder.

Couples therapy for reciprocal IPV

- No-violence contract
- Use of negotiated time-out tool
- Strategies to manage anger
- Treatment of comorbidity

Significant reduction in IPV occurs when comorbid alcoholism is successfully treated, and couples can enter couples treatment when the alcohol abuse/dependence is under control (26). Greater treatment involvement is associated with greater reduction in violence. Couples treatment consists of a sobriety contract, behavioral assignments, and relapse prevention (27). The behavioral assignments are aimed at increasing positive feelings, shared activities, and constructive criticism. At the end of treatment, each couple completes a continued recovery plan that is reviewed quarterly for 2 years. The reduction in IPV is mediated by reduced problem drinking and enhanced relationship functioning. This model is easy to incorporate into a clinical skill set.

For couples treatment, the PCSTF with an added IPV-psychoeducational module based on the work of Sandra Stith (28) is practical and easy to implement. The psychoeducational module uses a cognitive-behavioral approach and a negotiated time-out tool (29). The initial goals when meeting with the couple are as follows: agreeing that no violence will occur during treatment, understanding the history of violence in their relationship, learning the use of the time-out tool, and completing an assessment of family functioning. A problem list is generated during the assessment. Treatment involves ensuring that the changes the couple agrees to are actually carried out, as outlined in Chapter 9. A successful treatment of a couple using the PCSTF model is found in *Intimate Partner and Family Abuse: A Casebook of Gender Inclusive Therapy* (30).

Divorce

Divorce can be a positive solution to a destructive family situation. A conflict-ridden intact family can be more detrimental to its members than one that is stable even if reconstituted, although little empirical data exist on the long-term effects of divorce. In most studies, there is little control over the many confounding variables such as the age of parents and children, gender of the child, socioeconomic circumstances, social support, psychiatric and medical illnesses, quality of the postdivorce relationship, and the personalities of individuals in the family. As a result, prediction of predominant issues caused by divorce is best made on a case-by-case basis. It is important that a comprehensive assessment be made to establish an appropriate treatment plan.

Complex postdivorce families are common. These families may come to treatment with troubled, hurt, or angry accounts of family life and a sense that their circumstances are at odds with "life as it ought to be lived" (31). Most families respond to psychoeducation about the divorce process or interventions that work on negotiation of disagreements. Psychoeducation provides an understanding of the normal processes in divorce and the kinds of behaviors and feelings that typically unfold. The focus gradually shifts to helping both parents care for the children caught in parental conflict. The therapist uses data from divorce research to inform parents of the risks for children when parents are involved in protracted conflicts related to custody and visitation (32). Few parents fully appreciate the traumatic effect on children of ongoing parental conflict.

A subset of families with divorcing parents become high-conflict families and require more intensive treatment. These families engage in child custody disputes with children being used as pawns and others such as extended family members, friends, and lawyers becoming involved. High parental conflict is a powerful predictor of the negative effects of divorce for both children and adults (32, 33). In many states, programs have been developed to help with the resolution of conflicts, or at least to facilitate decision making with the goal of reducing lengthy court proceedings. A specific type of family therapy called integrative family therapy has been devised to target child custody and visitation (34). Many of the principles used in this model are similar to the PCSTF. For example, a detailed treatment contract is used that specifies who the participants in treatment are, frequency of visits, extent of court involvement, payment source, who has access to information, and how information will be shared with those outside the therapy. Intervention can occur across many levels. Psychoeducation is an important starting point. All family members are taught skills for respectfully disengaging from conflict, and children learn to respond to questions about the other parent with, "I am uncomfortable being in the middle of this." Integrative family therapy also utilizes mediation techniques to promote negotiation and improve problem solving. Anger management skills can be taught. If sessions become too intense, short breaks can be used to reduce affective tension. Unproductive sessions should be terminated.

Legal Issues

The process of reporting child, elder, and spousal abuse varies by state, so it is best to learn about specific legal and ethical knowledge in the state in which the physician practices. Informing families about the limits of confidentiality prior to seeing them can avoid conflict if the need for mandated reporting should arise. In cases in which the therapeutic relationship is significantly damaged by breaking confidentiality, the family may need to be referred to another clinician. It is best, however, to use the mandated reporting process as a means to strengthen the therapeutic alliance, for example, by informing the family that you can act as their advocate with the adult or child protective agency if they comply with treatment recommendations. This may be facilitated by allowing the family to be present in the room when you make the report by phone or by having a family member make the report as you provide support. Making a report of family violence can be an empowering act that helps family members begin to take control over their lives. It may also be helpful for victims of violence to watch others taking a stance against violent behavior by reporting it to authorities.

Conclusion

Families face a great variety of issues. While it is important to be knowledgeable about and sensitive to the kinds of problems families may encounter in different situations, it is also important to not approach families with preconceptions. There is no substitute for a comprehensive assessment of the family to determine, in concert with the family, what the problems are and what the family wants to do about them. It should be remembered that most families have strengths. Race and cultural difference can bring depth and richness to a family. The therapist should look for positive attributes. Regarding violence, couples with violent behavior can also have strengths (35); emphasizing positive attributes is therapeutic, as couples can be easily shamed when discussing their violence. At a minimum, couples can be commended for coming to treatment and acknowledging such a difficult problem as family violence. In summary, the important task is to engage the family and work with them to gain an understanding of their concerns, asking frequently for direction in this regard. The goal is always to work in a collaborative way with the family.

References

1. Knobloch-Fedders LM, Pinsof WM, Mann BJ: The formation of the therapeutic alliance in couple therapy. Fam Process 43:425–442, 2004

2. Knobloch-Fedders LM, Pinsof WM, Mann BJ: Therapeutic alliance and treatment progress in couple psychotherapy. J Marital Fam Ther 33:245–257, 2007

3. Garfield R: The therapeutic alliance in couples therapy: clinical considerations. Fam Process 43:457–465, 2004

4. Vasquez MJ: Cultural difference and the therapeutic alliance: an evidence-based analysis. Am Psychol 62:875–885, 2007

5. Eiser AR, Ellis G: Viewpoint: cultural competence and the African American experience with health care: the case for specific content in cross-cultural education. Acad Med 82:176–183, 2007

6. U.S. Department of Health and Human Services, Public Health Service, Office of the Surgeon General: Mental Health: Culture, Race, and Ethnicity. A Supplement to Mental Health: A Report of the Surgeon General (Executive Summary). Rockville, MD, U.S. Public Health Service, 2001

7. Dovidio JF, Gaertner SL, Kawakami K, et al: Why can't we just get along? Interpersonal biases and interracial distrust. Cult Divers Ethnic Minor Psychol 8:88–102, 2002

8. De Las Fuentes C: Latina/o America populations, in Clinical Practice With People of Color: A Guide to Becoming Culturally Competent. Edited by Constantine MG. New York, Teacher College, Columbia University, 2007, pp 46–60

9. Horowitz JA: Negotiating couplehood: the process of resolving the December dilemma among interfaith couples. Fam Process 38:303–323, 1999

10. Dyche L, Zayas LH: The value of curiosity and naiveté for the cross-cultural psychotherapist. Fam Process 34:389–399, 1995

11. Liddle B: Therapist sexual orientation, gender, and counseling practices as they relate to ratings of helpfulness by gay and lesbian clients. J Couns Psychol 43:394–401, 1996

12. MacDonald B: Issues in therapy with gay and lesbian couples. J Sex Marital Ther 24:165–190, 1998

13. Spitalnick JS, McNair LD: Couples therapy with gay and lesbian clients: an analysis of important clinical issues. J Sex Marital Ther 31:43–56, 2005 Jan-Feb
14. Greenan DE, Tunnell G: Couple Therapy With Gay Men. New York, Guilford, 2003
15. Laumann EO, Gagnon JH, Michael RT, et al: The Social Organization of Sexuality: Sexual Practices in the United States. Chicago, University of Chicago Press, 1994
16. Scheinkman M: Beyond the trauma of betrayal: reconsidering affairs in couples therapy. Fam Process 44:43–56, 2005
17. Atkins DC, Eldridge KA, Baucom DH, et al: Infidelity and behavioral couple therapy: optimism in the face of betrayal. J Consult Clin Psychol 73:144–150, 2005
18. Coop Gordon K, Baucom DH, Snyder DK: An integrative intervention for promoting recovery from extramarital affairs. J Marital Fam Ther 30:291–312, 2004
19. Tjaden P, Thoennes N: Prevalence, Incidence and Consequences of Violence Against Women: Findings From the National Violence Against Women Survey. Washington, DC, U.S. Department of Justice, 1998
20. Kessler RC, Monnar BE, Feurer ID, et al: Patterns and mental health predictors of domestic violence in the United States: results from the National Comorbidity Survey. Int J Law Psychiatry 24:487–508, 2002
21. Whitaker DJ, Haileyesus T, Swahn M, et al: Difference in frequency of violence and reported injury between relationships with reciprocal and nonreciprocal intimate partner violence. Am J Public Health 97:941–947, 2007
22. Archer J: Sex differences in aggression between heterosexual partners: a meta-analytic review. Psychol Bull 126:651–680, 2000
23. Langhinrichsen-Rohling D, Vivian J: Are bi-directionally violent couples mutually victimized? a gender-sensitive comparison. Viol Victims 9:107–124, 1994
24. Heru AM, Stuart GI, Rainey S, et al: Prevalence and severity of intimate partner violence and associations with family functioning and alcohol abuse in psychiatric inpatients with suicidal intent. J Clin Psychiatry 67:23–29, 2006
25. Bogard M, Mederos F: Battering and couples therapy: universal screening and selection of treatment modality. J Marital Fam Ther 25:291–312, 1999
26. O'Farrell TJ, Murphy CM, Stephan SH, et al: Partner violence before and after couples-based alcoholism treatment for male alcoholic patients: the role of treatment involvement and abstinence. J Consult Clin Psychol 72:202–217, 2004
27. O'Farrell T, Fals-Stewart W: Alcohol abuse. J Marital Fam Ther 29:121–146, 2003
28. Stith SM, McCollum EE, Rosen KH, et al: Multi-couples group treatment for domestic violence, in Comprehensive Handbook of Psychotherapy. Edited by Kaslow FW. New York, Wiley, 2004, pp 499–520

29. Rosen KH, Matheson JL, Stith SM, et al: Negotiated time-out: a deescalation tool for couples. J Marital Fam Ther 29:291–298, 2003

30. Heru AM: Intimate Partner and Family Abuse: A Casebook of Gender-Inclusive Therapy. New York, Springer, 2008

31. Bernstein AC: Re-visioning, restructuring, and reconciliation: clinical practice with complex post divorce families. Fam Process 46:67–78, 2007

32. Grych JH, Fincham FD, Jouriles EN, et al: Interparental conflict and child adjustment: testing the mediational role of appraisals in the cognitive-contextual framework. Child Dev 71:1648–1661, 2000

33. Amato PR: The "child of divorce" as a person prototype: bias in the recall of information about children in divorced families. J Marriage Fam 53:59–69, 1991

34. Lebow JL, Newcombrekart K: Integrative family therapy for high-conflict divorce with disputes over child custody and visitation. Fam Process 46:79–91, 2007

35. Heru AM, Stuart GI, Recupero PR: Family functioning in suicidal inpatients with intimate partner violence. Prim Care Companion J Clin Psychiatry 9:413–418, 2007

13

Training in Family Skills and Family Therapy

- All psychiatrists should be competent in general family skills, such as engaging families, developing a biopsychosocial formulation, and integrating family research findings into patient care.

- Every therapist should be able to identify family strengths and use these in treatment.

- For psychiatrists who wish to develop expertise in family therapy, understanding one family approach thoroughly is preferable to acquiring familiarity with many models.

Basic knowledge about family life stages is key to being able to understand families. The breadth and depth of family research informs clinical practice. This knowledge can be taught in didactic seminars throughout the residency program. This knowledge base fosters a family-friendly attitude in physicians who are then more open to the idea of including families in the assessment and treatment of patients.

The skills needed to work with families can be taught in a graded manner. Family medicine residency programs have taught family skills to their residents for many years (1) and use a schema easily adaptable to psychiatry. Five graded skill levels for residents are described, from being cordial to the family (level 1), to learning how to manage family interactions (levels 3–4), to being competent in family therapy (level 5). General family skills (levels 1–4) can be taught in the first and second years of residency. These skills include how to engage the family, assess the family, and work with the family on resolution of simple problems. Family therapy, a specific modality, and level 5 skills can be taught in the third and fourth years of training.

Levels for family training

- **Level 1:** Minimal emphasis on the family
- **Level 2:** Being open to engaging families and providing ongoing medical information and advice
- **Level 3:** Empathic listening, attentive to feelings, normalizing, identifying dysfunction, and supporting coping skills
- **Level 4:** Systematic assessment and planned intervention, skill in managing family interactions and recognizing dysfunctional patterns
- **Level 5:** Family therapy

Knowledge

Normal Family Development

Understanding normal family development and the family life cycle is basic to an understanding of families. Normal life transitions or family stages include courtship and marriage, birth or adoption of a child, adolescence and leaving home, midlife, retirement, and lastly illness or death of a family member. Patients often present with acute symptoms that occur when there is difficulty transitioning from one family life stage to another. At these transitions, the family task is to reorganize to include a new member, cope with the departure of a member, or accommodate someone in a new role. New family and individual skills may need to be learned. Knowledge of how a healthy family functions and manages transitions is therefore important (see Chapter 2). The commentary in scene 15 of the DVD reviews the difficulties a family has when one person is ill. Over the course of the assessment, the interviewing psychiatrist identifies that the illness of one family member may be one of the reasons why the daughter has moved back home and the son has moved away.

Family members often describe improvement in family functioning when a member becomes ill, expressing increased closeness and reward from caring. It is important to recognize and acknowledge family change that is beneficial. The dynamics of a family system can be described using the basic description of systemic change: "When one person becomes ill, then the other family members are affected." Similarly, if family change is to occur, then the whole family system must change. There also needs to be an understanding of common family situations, such as the effects of divorce, blended families, and single-parent families, as well as cultural and ethnic differences in family structure and functioning.

Family Research

Introducing family research as early as possible in the training process helps to promote family-friendly attitudes. Family research provides the rationale for involving families in assessment and treatment. Family research shows that working with families improves outcome for patients with physical illnesses (2) and psychiatric illnesses (3) as well as for children with psychiatric illness (4) (see Chapter 3). Family involvement in patient care is recommended in the American Psychiatric Association's Practice Guidelines for many disorders (5, 6, 7). The guidelines recommend early family involvement and outline the evidence of the efficacy of marital or family therapy for specific diagnoses.

Skills

General Family Skills

There is a recent emphasis on teaching residents how to interact effectively with families in all treatment settings. This change has occurred in conjunction with the Accreditation Council for Graduate Medical Education (ACGME) residency expectations that residents demonstrate competency in six core areas: patient care, medical knowledge, interpersonal and communication skills, systems-based practice, professionalism, and practice-based learning and improvement. In psychiatry, families are discussed in five of these six core competencies. For example, in interpersonal and communication skills, residents are expected to demonstrate an ability to educate patients, their families, and professionals about medical, psychosocial, and behavioral issues. Residents are expected to develop a working alliance with patients and their families and to ensure that the patient and family have understood the communication. The Family Committee of the Group for the Advancement of Psychiatry (GAP), a psychiatric think tank, has developed a set of general family skills for residents based on the ACGME core competencies (8). The GAP criteria provide clear and measurable expectations for residents to meet the family component of these core competencies (see Appendix 13–1 at the end of this chapter).

Beginning residents experience working with families as "messy" and need guidance in how to develop goals for a family meeting and to manage family interactions. They may see few psychiatrists working with families and develop the idea that family work is not in the domain of the psychiatrist. Good physician role models who understand a systems perspective and practice a biopsychosocial approach to patient care provide the best supervision for residents at the beginning of their residency. They do not need to be family therapists. Each clinical setting provides an opportunity for general family skills to be taught (9). It is also helpful for practicing psychiatrists to be exposed to colleagues who involve families, on a regular basis, in the care of their patients. Familiarity with the process and normalization of the practice, especially if it is seen to be helpful, can go a long way to encouraging similar approaches by others.

Psychiatric Inpatient Unit

The inpatient unit is the ideal place to begin resident training in family skills. Families are frequently involved in hospitalization and discharge planning, so residents can be socialized from the beginning of training to treat the families' contributions with respect. Families are more likely to agree to a meeting when a crisis is at hand or when there is concern about safety. Patients and families are also more open to the possibility of change as their usual ways of coping have not worked. Residents can work independently with families (after appropriate preparatory training), but faculty should be available to participate in meetings with contentious families and with inexperienced residents. It is a mistake to expect residents or psychiatrists who are just learning family interventions to meet with families before receiving training. There is a good likelihood that they will encounter difficulties and anxiety along with feelings of inadequacy and helplessness. These feelings make it more likely that they will not involve families in the care of their patients in the future. It is far preferable to have the physician participate in some didactic presentations, watch someone else conduct family meetings, and then conduct them independently.

Family skills with inpatient families

- Being able to conduct an interview with the patient present, regardless of the diagnosis
- Appreciating and validating the concerns and emotional reactions of family members to the patient's illness and hospitalization
- Taking seriously the family's concerns about too-early discharge or inadequate follow-up plans and their questions about caregiving and further emergency care
- Ensuring opportunities for family psychoeducation related to the illness of the patient, treatment options, both pharmacological and psychosocial, expected treatment, and prognosis
- Ensuring that family members learn about the need for social support, respite, and self-care and about family support organizations such as the National Alliance on Mental Illness and the Depression and Bipolar Support Alliance

---

Psychiatric Emergency Room

Patients brought to the emergency room may be incapable of giving an accurate history. Family members are often involved in the emergence of the crisis and may be anxious, angry, or emotionally distraught. In these situations, residents can develop skills in history gathering from multiple sources. Psychiatrists should learn how to develop a therapeutic alliance with the family (interpersonal and communication skills), show respect for culturally diverse patients and their families (professionalism), and educate the patient and the family concerning the system of care (systems-based practice). Supervision in this setting can focus on the support and struggles of patients' family members and guidance about managing the family in a crisis. It is also an opportunity to learn about problems of access, adequacy, and coordination of resources.

Outpatient Clinic

Patients come to the outpatient clinic for a variety of reasons, and it is the task of the physician to evaluate the extent to which involving the family is necessary. Family members are frequently involved with patients, for example, becoming responsible for medication compliance or managing side effects of medications or therapy. If the patient is seriously ill, family members must manage the crisis. Meeting with the family as soon as possible is therefore recommended. Psychiatrists may not want to take the patient's first "no" as a final decision. In the same way that one would not accept a "no" to medications without continued discussion, the psychiatrist with a patient in serious distress or with a relational problem should feel confident in persisting with the position that involving the family on some level is part of treatment.

Family psychoeducation in the outpatient setting includes education about course of the illness, the role and side effects of medication, agreement about what constitutes a relapse or crisis, when the physician should be contacted, and whether or not the family has a role in medication monitoring. Regarding confidentiality, the physician distinguishes between private individual session content and the case management issues described above, which can be shared. In addition, particularly with impaired young adults living at home and unable to work, an agreement about family rules, especially about the structure of the patient's day, alcohol or drug use, and finances, is helpful.

Patients who seek outpatient psychotherapy may refuse a family consultation. The physician should assess whether the presenting or associated problems are relational in nature and whether involving the family might improve the patient's outcome. For example, if the patient is in a committed relationship and is experiencing relational problems, a couples consultation, done either by the treating physician or a colleague, may be critical to determining whether couples therapy would be useful. Patients often present for individual therapy for relational issues such as divorce without first mentioning to their partners that they are dissatisfied and want relational change. Even well-functioning patients typically present a one-sided view of relational issues, and the treating physician who sees the patient and partner together (even for a single assessment session) gains a healthy respect for the amount of information missed by hearing only one side of the issue.

Substance Abuse Clinic

Outpatient treatment of addiction should be family based if the patient is living with family members or is in touch with their family who continues to support them. Patients with substance dependence will minimize their substance use, so corroborating information from the family is useful. Families also need clear guidelines about how to interact with the recovering patient, education about addiction, guidance on how to set limits while continuing to be supportive, and strong encouragement to attend Al-Anon, Nar-Anon, or other appropriate groups. Rather than apportioning blame, the dilemmas of partners of patients with alcohol dependence need to be explored (10). Behavioral couples therapy is a successful treatment for patients with alcoholism and reduces intimate partner violence (11) as well as improves the health of children of substance-dependent fathers (12).

Psychosomatic Medicine (Consultation/Liaison) Service

On the psychosomatic medicine service, a family member's history is often critical in determining whether a patient's symptoms occurred before or after hospitalization and medical treatment and whether the medical regimen is contributing to the symptoms. With chronic medical illness, caregiver burden may need specific attention. Patients may be in conflict with their relatives or staff about medical care, and psychiatrists can be called to negotiate or mediate between care providers, the family, and the patient. There is tremendous opportunity for residents to learn how to take a good history, develop an understanding of the conflicts, and help negotiate a treatment plan.

In recently developed medical problems, families are faced with learning to cope and adapt to a family member's illness. Family roles may change drastically, dealing with medical systems may produce feelings of helplessness or rage, and family routines and habits are invariably disrupted (13). Psychiatric consultation with key family members near the time of initial diagnosis and at major nodal points during the course of the illness (e.g., rehospitalization, recurrence or progression of the illness, transfer to rehabilitation or hospice) can facilitate the treatment process and support the family unit in a time of crisis. Convening families in this context is not difficult as family members typically visit their hospitalized member. This requires flexibility, a willingness to meet with families in the late afternoon or early evening after typical work hours, or a willingness to conduct rounds during visiting hours.

Goals of psychosomatic family meeting

- To emphasize that all family members are affected by the strains and challenges of living with a major medical illness and to address the immediate emotional and practical needs of the patient and family members, such as guilt, shame, helplessness, and the reactivation of old family conflicts around illness decision making.

- To facilitate communication around illness and treatment-related issues and decisions. Inability of family members to speak to each other, particularly about death and dying, often makes these processes painful and stunts family growth for years to come.

- To help the family understand the illness in longitudinal and developmental terms. While this is true in psychiatric illness as well, physical illness alters the family landscape in very specific ways in terms of role change and grief within the family.

- To understand the cultural and spiritual beliefs that guide the family. This is essential to fostering culturally sensitive collaborative care and helping the family make meaning of the illness experience.

Family Therapy Training

Throughout this book the general outline of the McMaster Model of Family Functioning is used to describe an approach to families. In this section, the training associated with the Problem-Centered Systems Therapy of the Family (PCSTF) is described. This is the treatment model associated with the McMaster Model assessment as described in Chapters 4 and 9.

Family therapy training consists of conceptual, perceptual, and executive skills. Conceptual skills include learning the definitions, concepts, and theories related to family systems models as well as the theory, concepts, and definitions of how a family functions according to the McMaster Model. Perceptual skills include the ability to perceive the data, that is, to accurately identify family behaviors and interactions, and then relate them to the conceptual model. Understanding a clinical case and translating the data into a conceptual framework is a key part of training. Executive skills include those needed to apply treatment concepts according to the PCSTF.

Training occurs best in small groups of four to six trainees. The feedback given to trainees is substantial, and limiting the number of participants provides comfort and ease with the process. For maximum benefit from supervision, trainees should bring tapes of family sessions for review and discussion. Training may take 12–14 months to learn and develop basic comfort with the model and to have enough practice with live families to gain a sense of mastery.

Training Sessions: Months 1–3

The overview sessions for the first part of the training include didactic material and family videotapes of the McMaster approach. The objectives for the first sessions are to provide an introduction to the six dimensions of the McMaster Model and the macro stages of the PCSTF. Conceptual skills training at this stage involves small group discussions on the concepts associated with the McMaster Model, family systems thinking, family development, and family crises. The dimensions of the McMaster Model are reviewed, including problem solving, communication, role allocation, affective responsiveness, affective involvement, and behavior control. After trainees understand the concepts, they need to develop perceptual skills, that is, be able to identify and label them in real life. This stage of the training makes use of videotapes, DVDs, and direct observations of family sessions. Role-playing may be used with residents playing family members in a simulated family scenario.

Training Sessions: Months 4–6

Training now focuses on the developing skills necessary to complete a comprehensive family assessment. During this part of training, the conceptual and perceptual skills are refined and reinforced, and executive skills are introduced. After one or two role-plays as a therapist, trainees become actively involved in seeing families for assessment. The trainee's work situations, level of experience, and ability are taken into account in assigning cases. Trainees may do a partial assessment (i.e., the orientation and one or two dimensions) with the family before attempting a full assessment. Alternatively, one trainee may be responsible for orienting the family and identifying the presenting problems while another trainee may be responsible for assessing some of the other dimensions. Sessions should be videotaped to provide feedback to the trainees. Audiotaped sessions are an alternative. These tapes are reviewed in the small group supervisory sessions.

Training Sessions: Months 6–12

Once a trainee has a reasonable grasp of the assessment process, he or she is able to begin work in completing a full comprehensive family interview. To establish competency, the trainee should fully assess at least two families and obtain feedback from the supervisor. At this point, the trainee is ready to initiate family treatment according to the PCSTF. The supervision at this advanced stage of training is concentrated on executive skill development. Trainees videotape their family therapy sessions for feedback from the supervisor and fellow trainees in the small group seminars. In review of the videotapes, the following key points are kept in mind for feedback to the trainee: Are the stages as defined by the PCSTF being followed? Have the presenting problems been delineated and the tasks negotiated as they relate to the McMaster Model dimensions? Has the trainee recognized and utilized family transactions and interactions in his or her treatment interventions? Has the trainee intervened appropriately if the family did not follow through with tasks, had difficulty with the tasks, or had broken their contract? Is the trainee able to discuss and manage issues related to engaging, assessing, treating, terminating, and providing referrals for follow-up care for their families?

Training is completed when trainees have shown competence in assessing and treating at least three families. Trainees demonstrate their competency in treating families by engaging the family and keeping them in treatment, identifying transactional patterns within the family, successfully contracting with families for change, dealing with resistance appropriately, and maintaining clarity of treatment goals.

Supervision

Training in general family skills can be given by any psychiatrist with an understanding of families, systems, and a biopsychosocial approach to patient care. Training in family therapy needs to be given by a physician or an allied mental health professional proficient in that model of family therapy. There are many models of family therapy, but as with individual therapy, trainees should be encouraged to master the use of one model. Outcome studies are the same for all family therapies regardless of theoretical orientation in the same way that outcome is similar for all individual psychotherapies regardless of theoretical orientation (14).

Supervision issues for general family skills

- Treat family meetings as a normative part of patient care
- Acknowledge challenges in meeting with families
- View the family system as the unit of care
- Engage each family member
- Avoid taking sides
- Be aware of trainee's own family dynamic affecting interactions
- Begin family meeting with an orientation
- Include diagnosis and treatment plan discussion in family meeting

---

General Skills Supervision

Supervisors in general family skills can support trainee efforts in arranging a family meeting, even if the patient is reluctant, and in making family meetings a normative part of care. Meeting with families and documenting discussion of safety issues including side effects of medications are good risk management strategies (15). General family issues for residents and supervisors to discuss in supervision include family life cycle stages, the effect of illness on family communication and functioning, family factors contributing to the patient's illness, caregiver burden, and psychoeducation. Supervisors can encourage, demonstrate, or participate in initial family interviewing and provide planning and postmeeting supervision when the trainee is able to manage the session alone.

Challenges trainees face when working with families need to be understood and addressed; otherwise, training is frustrating (16). First, an understanding of the nature of the therapeutic relationship between the psychiatrist and the family is necessary before proceeding. The relationship with the family is different from a relationship with an individual patient. The relationship is with a family system, which means that the trainee must gain an understanding of how the family system works: is it a rigid or flexible system, does it tolerate difference, are there acceptable and unacceptable behaviors?

For the beginning trainee, the first task is to try to engage all family members in the process of a meeting and to avoid being pulled into an alliance with one particular member against the others. This alignment often happens when the trainee has worked extensively with the identified patient, who may have hostile or ambivalent opinions about his or her family members. This situation may occur with an adolescent in a developmental struggle with parents or between partners where the nonpatient is perceived as controlling or dominating. The beginning trainee must beware of rescue fantasies that might entail siding with one family member against another. The trainee may be more sympathetic toward his or her patient and side with the patient against the rest of the family, especially if there are facts in dispute. The trainee may have particular feelings about a specific family member that may remind the trainee of one of his or her own family members.

Trainees may have specific difficulties when working with families that resonate with their own childhood experiences so that trainees who have histories of abuse, neglect, alcoholism, or psychotic parents may want to avoid family interaction. Trainees who have no siblings are often at a loss with large families, and trainees who have had no experience with other cultures might get very flustered by different family systems. Older couples whose children have recently left home may want to draw a trainee into the family system to replace their recent loss. It is important to acknowledge that trainees can be drawn into a family system and may occupy a familiar role. The supervisor can remind trainees that their own personal experience of their own family affects their perception of the patient's family and then provide a safe forum for discussion.

Within a family system, all family members need to be engaged. Any family conflicts can be discussed, and the family can agree on where each member stands vis-à-vis the conflict. Gunderson (17) commented that when he actually met the family members of his borderline personality disorder patients, they were not the terrible people his patients had described. From then on, he included the families in treatment and has developed a psychoeducational program that helps both patients and family members.

A family meeting begins with an orientation as to the purpose of the meeting. The orientation should include the explanation that each person will have a limited time to talk because it is important to hear from everyone. Trainees can explain in a respectful way that they may need to interrupt to allow everyone time to speak. As the meeting progresses, the trainees can refer back to their previous statement that they might have to ask a family member to stop talking. This reduces potential feelings of shame or anger at being interrupted and allows the trainee to remain in control of the meeting. The meeting also should include a discussion of diagnosis, the results of current assessments, and a tentative treatment plan.

Trainee concerns

- The family is causing the patient's problems.
- There's no time to meet with families.
- I can't determine what the family wants.
- I don't know what's wrong yet.
- The family is hostile and demanding.
- I feel outnumbered and don't understand what is happening.
- I don't understand the family's culture or background.
- No one expects residents to see families.
- I'm not sure whether to see patient and family together or separately.
- What about the patient's confidentiality?

Common Trainee Concerns

"The family is causing the patient's problems." Psychiatry has a history of blaming the family for causing psychiatric illness and using pejorative labeling, such as the "schizophrenogenic" mother (18). A beginning trainee's desire to be empathic toward the patient may unwittingly ostracize family members who are often a focus for the patient's anger. It is important to ask trainees to put themselves in the shoes of the family: "If this were your family member, how would you like to be treated, and what would you need to know?" "What has transpired over the past years?" Thinking about the family's perspective helps the trainee engage with the family in a more empathic way. Trainees need to be reminded of the fallacy equating correlation with causation. It is often unclear whether family dysfunction contributes to or is a result of a patient's psychopathology.

"There's no time to meet with families."   Meeting with families improves patient compliance (19, 20), strengthens the alliance between patient and physician (21), sets the stage for future problem solving (22), and has a positive influence on patient outcome (23). It is therefore cost-effective in terms of time and resources to meet with families. Stating that there is no time to meet with the family may be a way of avoiding the family, especially if the family is perceived as angry or demanding or is expressing high levels of emotion, which can be difficult for the trainee to tolerate.

"What does the family want?"   Family members usually see themselves as advocates and want to be involved (24). Families may express a sense of failure as they acknowledge their inability to resolve family problems and may express guilt or blame themselves for their relative's illness. In a family meeting, family members may be anxious as they anticipate being discussed, criticized, blamed, and confronted. Children may fear being punished, getting their parents in trouble, or being caught in loyalty conflicts. Families state that they do not want lengthy and intensive interventions but rather family care that focuses on building rapport and communication with mental health professionals (25). Families therefore express several needs: to be included in the care of their relative, to be understood, and to be respected as family members who are doing their best.

"But I don't know what's wrong yet!"   Physicians may avoid meeting with the family if they do not have a definitive diagnosis and treatment plan because they do not want to be seen as uncertain or incompetent. Being straightforward with the family about the need to gather more information is acceptable to most families. Meeting with the family for a short time to explain the process will help engage the family and establish a collaborative relationship. This in turn will make it more likely that the family will be open to providing information that can be very helpful in gaining a better understanding of the presenting problems. The willingness of the trainee to reach out to a family is reassuring to the family and is seen as supportive and caring.

"The family is hostile and demanding."   The hostile family, if ignored, is likely to become more demanding. The trainee is encouraged to think about what it must be like for the family to have someone hospitalized. Do they feel responsible and blame themselves? Do they feel helpless and worried that their relative has a major mental illness? Is their list of questions an attempt to gain some control and reduce their fears? Are they advocating for their relative? What do they understand about the process of hospitalization?

"I feel outnumbered and don't understand what is happening." Trainees avoid families because they perceive themselves as unskilled. Trainees report feeling anxious in a family meeting because "there are too many dynamics and emotions flying around," there is "difficulty keeping track" of the flow of dialogue, and they feel unable to incorporate the multiple perspectives of the various family members. Providing structure to a family meeting reduces dynamic interactions and gives the trainee a road map for the meeting (16, 26).

"I don't understand the family's culture or background." It is helpful to be knowledgeable about a particular culture, but frequently descriptions do not "fit." There is therefore benefit in presenting oneself as naive and open to learning from the family about their culture and family structure (27). This attitude of respect, acceptance, and willingness to learn helps the family feel more at ease in the interview.

"No one expects residents to see families." The resident may perceive the social worker or the marriage and family therapist as the person to meet with the family. Medical family therapists are becoming part of the team in many different specialties because they are cheaper, more attentive to patients and families, and increasingly used by managed care to bridge the gap between the medical profession and the family's needs (28). It is a major tenet of this book that competent physicians must be able to work with families to be leaders in the mental health field.

"I'm not sure whether to see the patient and family together or separately." The trainee often realizes that there are relationship issues with the patient and then wonders whether to refer the couple/family elsewhere or see them themselves. Another common scenario is when the trainee is confused about what is going on with the patient and wants to bring in other family members to see if they can provide helpful information. In both these scenarios, it is acceptable to bring family members in as part of the assessment of the patient. It can be explained to family members that a family assessment usually takes one or two sessions and is considered part of a routine comprehensive assessment.

After the assessment, the trainee and couple/family can decide whether they wish to engage in treatment. If family treatment is indicated, who should carry out the treatment? This depends on several factors, such as the trainee's therapeutic relationship with the patient, the perceptions of the family, and the trainee's skill level. The psychiatrist might find it hard to work in a systemic way if the relationship with the patient is intense and has been ongoing for a period of time. The patient may also find it difficult to share the psychiatrist with other family members and may be fearful that confidential information might be inadvertently shared or influence the treatment. The patient may feel that treatment would not be successful if the family perceived the therapist to be taking sides rather than impartial. The family members similarly may feel that impartiality would be impossible if they shared the patient's psychiatrist. Fairness has been identified as one of five preconditions for change in couples therapy (29). If the psychiatrist is unable to establish an atmosphere of fairness, then working with the family will be ineffective. If a patient has severe psychopathology, then the psychiatrist might benefit from working with a team of professionals to prevent burnout. In these cases, referral to another therapist is justified. (Also see Chapter 10 for a fuller description of this issue.)

"**What about patient confidentiality?**" Trainees frequently ask about how to handle confidential information. As a general rule, it is best to foster an open relationship with all members of the family and to encourage the sharing of information. However, sometimes patients will say that they do not want certain information given to their family, and sometimes family members may ask to talk with the physician without the patient being present.

The desire to talk confidentially with the psychiatrist should always be considered to be a helpful gesture on the part of the family member. It may relate to questions about the best way to convey information and a desire to protect the patient as much as possible. For example, the parents of a young male patient were concerned about their son's psychiatric diagnosis and the meaning of his behavior in the context of the family's history of Huntington's disease. After consultation with the neurologist, it was considered best to defer discussion of this history with the patient.

Sometimes, however, motives may be misguided. For example, a young married woman stated to the psychiatrist, prior to the meeting with her husband, that she had a secret stash of medications at home that was her backup suicide plan. She explicitly forbade the psychiatrist from disclosing this information to her husband. The psychiatrist did not want to openly betray her trust but stated that her husband should know about it. The patient adamantly refused and became hostile to the psychiatrist. At the family meeting, the psychiatrist gave the patient ample opportunity to discuss this plan, for example, "Do you ever feel unsafe at home?" "Do you have any suicide plans?" The patient refused to divulge the presence of her secret stash. Last-ditch efforts included comments like "Do you have anything you wish to tell your husband about your safety?" The husband then questioned the psychiatrist about the persistent questions regarding safety. The psychiatrist deflected the question back to his wife, saying "I think you should be directing that question to your wife." The wife was furious but did divulge the presence of a secret stash of medications. Medico-legally the psychiatrist had acted appropriately, yet maintained the patient's confidentiality in the presence of a potential but not imminent risk. Ultimately, however, the patient could no longer work with the psychiatrist. If information is shared individually, it is useful to ask if that information can be shared with the whole family because secrets can perpetuate mistrust and perception of collusion between the psychiatrist and the family member.

This patient with long-standing characterological deficits failed to engage with the psychiatrist because of the perceived breach of confidentiality. However, it is important to note that the family meeting had possibly been instrumental in ensuring her survival.

Assessment of Trainees

Knowledge

A trainee's knowledge can be assessed by documentation of attendance at seminars or completion of assigned readings. In practice, trainees need to show that they can answer questions about family functioning, such as: What is the family's developmental stage? What are the family's strengths? What are the dimensions of family functioning that should be assessed? Knowledge about a specific model of assessment and treatment is best accomplished in small group supervisory settings. The application of knowledge can be assessed during case discussion or chart-stimulated recall. The resident's understanding of how family factors enhanced a particular treatment outcome or how a particular family interview was crucial in managing a patient within the family system can be discussed. Examples can be included in portfolios and case logs.

Attitude

A trainee's positive attitude toward families is reflected in a willingness to engage the family in the assessment and treatment process. Attitude is also reflected in the ability of the trainee to find families to work with. Simple documentation of reaching out to families by telephone and by arranging family meetings is adequate for trainees training to level 2 (openness to engaging families and providing ongoing medical information and advice). At more advanced levels, the trainee can demonstrate a willingness to proactively seek out family strengths, engage difficult families, and provide family psychoeducational material as a routine part of patient care. Helping the patient and family understand the benefit of family-oriented care and providing appropriate research data display a real understanding of family-oriented care.

Skills

Trainees report that the best learning experiences occur when they have hands-on supervision with cases in which a good outcome is likely (30). A good outcome occurs when the trainee and family case are matched in terms of level of difficulty. This judgment is a basic skill of a good supervisor.

Assessing family skills must answer the questions: Can the trainee engage the family, understand their concerns, assess family functioning and communicate a family-friendly formulation to the family, provide psychoeducation regarding treatment, and carry out family-focused treatment?

Assessment tools are available for the McMaster Model and the PCSTF, including the McMaster PCSTF Adherence Scale, McMaster PCSTF Competence Scale, McMaster Family Functioning Concept Test, and McMaster Family Functioning Percept Test (31). Assessment of specific family skills will depend on the trainee's year of training and the site of assessment (e.g., inpatient, outpatient). At levels 3 and 4, more extensive evaluation is necessary by observing and providing feedback at family interviews. Assessment forms for family therapy trainees are outlined in this chapter's Appendix 13–2.

Conclusion

Young practicing psychiatrists state that family skills were the least taught during their residency and among the skills most needed after graduation (30). When trainees receive early exposure to families, they understand the importance of working with families. Watching their supervisors working with families and understanding the research that validates the inclusion of families in patient care are also important ingredients of good training. Teaching general family skills early in the trainee's professional career provides the best chance that the trainee will integrate these skills into his or her professional work as a matter of routine. Trainees with family skills can use these skills in other situations in which an ability to use a systems perspective is important, such as working with nurses, social workers, and an interdisciplinary team. Physicians are often asked to be leaders, and family skills are invaluable in this regard.

References

1. Doherty WJ: Boundaries between patient and family education and family therapy. Fam Relat 44:353–358, 1995
2. Campbell TL: The effectiveness of family interventions for physical disorders. J Marital Fam Ther 29:263–281, 2003
3. Heru AM: Family psychiatry: from research to practice. Am J Psychiatry 163:962–968, 2006
4. Diamond G, Josephson AJ: Family-based treatment research: a 10-year update. Am Acad Child Adolesc Psychiatry 44:872–887, 2005
5. American Psychiatric Association Work Group on Depressive Disorder: Practice guideline for the treatment of patients with depressive disorder (revision). Am J Psychiatry 157 (4 suppl):1–45, 2000
6. American Psychiatric Association Work Group on Schizophrenia: Practice guideline for the treatment of patients with bipolar disorder (revision). Am J Psychiatry 159 (4 suppl):1–50, 2002
7. American Psychiatric Association Work Group on Schizophrenia: Practice guideline for the treatment of patients with schizophrenia, 2nd edition. Am J Psychiatry 161 (2 suppl):1–56, 2004
8. Berman EM, Heru A, Grunebaum H, et al: Group for the Advancement of Psychiatry Committee on the Family: Family skills for general psychiatry residents: meeting ACGME core competency requirements. Acad Psychiatry 30:69–78, 2006
9. Berman EM, Heru A, Grunebaum H, et al: Group for the Advancement of Psychiatry Committee on the Family: Family-oriented patient care through the residency training cycle. Acad Psychiatry 32:111–118, 2008
10. Rotunda RJ, West L, O'Farrell TJ: Enabling behavior in a clinical sample of alcohol-dependent clients and their partners. J Subst Abuse Treat 26:269–276, 2004

11. O'Farrell T, Fals-Stewart W: Alcohol abuse. J Marital Fam Ther 29:121–146, 2003

12. Andreas JB, O'Farrell TJ, Fals-Stewart W: Does individual treatment for alcoholic fathers benefit their children? A longitudinal assessment. J Consult Clin Psychol 74:191–198, 2006

13. Rolland JS: Families, Illness and Disability: An Integrative Treatment Model. New York, Basic Books, 1994

14. Parker G, Fletcher K: Treating depression with evidence-based psychotherapies: a critique of the evidence. Acta Psychiatr Scand 115:352–359, 2007

15. Recupero PR: Risk management and the family, in Working With Families of Psychiatric Inpatients. Edited by Heru AM, Drury L. Baltimore, MD, Johns Hopkins University Press, 2007, pp 139–148

16. Heru AM, Drury L: Working With Families of Psychiatric Inpatients. Baltimore, MD, Johns Hopkins University Press, 2007

17. Gunderson JG, Berkowitz C, Ruiz-Sancho A: Families of borderline patients: a psychoeducational approach. Bull Menninger Clin 61:446–457, 1997

18. Neil J: Whatever became of the schizophrenogenic mother? Am J Psychother 44:499–505, 1990

19. Baird MA, Doherty WJ: Risks and benefits of a family systems approach to medical care. Fam Process 22:396–403, 1990

20. McDaniel SH, Campbell TL, Seaburn DB: Family-Oriented Primary Care: A Manual for Medical Providers. New York, Springer-Verlag, 1990

21. Marvel MK, Doherty WJ, Weiner E: Medical interviewing by exemplary family physicians. J Fam Practice 47:343–348, 1998

22. Lang F, Marvel K, Sanders D: Interviewing when family members are present. Am Fam Physician 65:1351–1354, 2002

23. Brown JB, Brett P, Stewart MA: Roles and influences of people who accompany patients on visits to doctor. Can Fam Physician 444:1644–1650, 1998

24. Leavey G, King M, Cole E: First-onset psychotic illness: patients' and relatives' satisfaction with services. Br J Psychiatry 170:53–57, 1997

25. Rose LE, Mallinson RK, Walton-Moss B: Barriers to family care in psychiatric settings. J Nurs Scholarship 36:39–47, 2004

26. Heru AM: Basic family skills for an inpatient psychiatrist: meeting ACGME core competency requirements. Fam Sys Health 22:216–227, 2004

27. Dyche L, Zayas LH: The value of curiosity and naiveté for the cross-cultural psychotherapist. Fam Process 34:389–399, 1995

28. Van Heden H: Training for collaboration: a study of medical family interns. Diss Abstr Int Sect B: Sci Engineering 62:1103, 2001

29. Christensen LL, Russell CS, Miller RB: The process of change in couples therapy: a qualitative investigation. J Marital Fam Ther 24:177–188, 1989

30. Gutman HA, Feldman RB, Engelsmann F, et al: The relationship between psychiatrists' couple and family therapy training experience and their subsequent practice profile. J Marital Fam Ther 25:31–41, 1999
31. Ryan CE, Epstein N, Keitner GI, et al: Evaluating and Treating Families: The McMaster Approach. New York, Routledge Taylor & Francis Group, 2005

Appendix 13–1

Group for the Advancement of Psychiatry (GAP) Proposal for Specific Family Systems Competencies

Knowledge

The resident is expected to demonstrate knowledge of family factors as they relate to psychiatric and nonpsychiatric disorders, based on scientific literature and standards of practice. The resident is expected to demonstrate knowledge of the following:

1. Basic concepts of systems, applicable to families, multidisciplinary teams in clinical settings, and medical/government organizations affecting the patient and doctor.
2. Couple and family development over the life cycle and the importance of multigenerational patterns.
3. Principles of adaptive and maladaptive relational functioning in family life: family organization, communication, problem solving, and emotional regulation.
4. Family strengths, resilience, and vulnerability.
5. How age, gender, class, culture, and spirituality affect family life.
6. The variety of family forms (single parent, stepfamily, same-sex parents, etc.).
7. How the family affects and is affected by psychiatric and nonpsychiatric disorders. This includes specific information regarding the impact of parental psychiatric illness on children.
8. Special issues in family life, including loss, divorce and remarriage, immigration, illness, secrets, affairs, violence, alcohol and substance abuse, sexuality (including gay, lesbian, bisexual, and transgender issues).
9. Relationship of families to larger systems (e.g., schools, work, health care systems, government agencies).

Attitudes

The attitudes held and demonstrated by the competent resident are empathy, curiosity, and respect for all family members. The resident must accept differences in perspectives on the problem and solution and understand that, in families, there is no ultimate truth. This is demonstrated by:

1. Allowing each family member to describe the presenting problem.
2. Identifying and acknowledging strengths and prior attempts at problem solving.
3. Acknowledging realistic limitations while maintaining an attitude of hopefulness.
4. Showing balanced concern for each member of the family and his or her point of view.
5. Working collaboratively with families and seeing them as allies.

Skills

The resident should demonstrate reasonable ability to conduct a family interview and to complete an assessment and formulation that include family factors. Operational skills include:

1. Identify family members and other relevant persons in larger systems who are involved with the patient's current functioning. In adult residency programs, this might include parents, spouses, partners, adults or children, extended family, staff in health care and other systems.
2. Meet with patient's significant family members and be able to deal with reluctance on the part of patient or family to meet.
3. Foster a therapeutic alliance with all family members by instilling feelings of trust, openness, and rapport.
4. In an assessment interview, the resident should:
   a. Elicit each family member's perspective of the presenting problem.
   b. Obtain a family history, including strengths, stressors, and repeating intergenerational patterns of behavior or illness. The ability to construct a genogram and a timeline is helpful in this process.
   c. Elicit the family's culture, class, etc., and describe how these affect their response to the patient and his or her illness and treatment.
   d. Identify and assess the emotional climate, family organization, and interactional problem solving as described by the Global Assessment of Relational Functioning (GARF). Include the GARF score in assessment.

    e. Be aware of personal feelings in relation to family members and be able to tolerate and work effectively in the presence of intense affects, especially when directed at the resident.

    f. Elicit strengths, competencies, and resources of couples and families so that they become useful and effective allies in treatment.

5. Following the interview, the resident should be able to:

    a. Integrate the impact of current relational functioning into the case formulation.

    b. Present the case formulation and, if appropriate, psychoeducation to the family in a frame that is respectful, culturally acceptable, and comprehensible.

    c. Involve the family members in collaborative treatment planning. Support the family in resolving differences of opinions with family members regarding treatment.

    d. Make recommendations for interventions, which may include other members of the system, such as the treatment of depression in the spouse.

For each of the core competencies, the level of expertise is as follows:

1. In patient care, the resident must demonstrate the ability to perform and document an adequate sociocultural and family history and to formulate a treatment plan that includes sociocultural aspects.

2. In medical knowledge, the resident needs to demonstrate knowledge of the experience, meaning, and explanation of the illness for the patient and the family. In addition, the resident should understand the family factors associated with specific illnesses, such as genetic implications, caregiver burden associated with chronic illness, and the normal developmental stages of the family.

3. In interpersonal and communication skills, the resident must demonstrate the ability to listen to and understand family members, communicate effectively about the treatment plan with the patient and family, and provide patient/family education. These communications should be jargon free and geared to the family's educational/intellectual level and be respectful of the family's cultural, ethnic, and economic background and identity and their impact on the experience, meaning, and evaluation of

the illness. Residents need to demonstrate the ability to develop a working alliance with the patients and their families.

4. In practice-based learning and improvement, the resident must demonstrate the ability to assess the generalizability or applicability of research findings to specific patients and the families.

5. In professionalism, the resident must demonstrate respect for culturally diverse patients and their families and be able to differentiate their own experiences from those of the family.

6. In systems-based practice, the resident should be able to educate the patients and their families concerning systems of care.

Source. Reprinted from Berman EM, Heru AM, Grunebaum H, et al: "Family Skills for General Psychiatry Residents: Meeting ACGME Core Competency Requirements." *Academic Psychiatry* 30:69–78, 2006. Used with permission.

Appendix 13–2

Assessment Forms for Family Therapy Trainees

A. Family Skills

Please rate as appropriate on a scale of 1–5, with 3 as expected level of performance.

The resident is able to:

Identify the role of family in presenting problem	1 2 3 4 5
Identify the family's developmental stage/transition	1 2 3 4 5
Identify any pertinent cultural/special situations	1 2 3 4 5
Identify the family's strengths and resources	1 2 3 4 5
Be supportive, respectful, and collaborative	1 2 3 4 5
Show balanced concern for each person's point of view	1 2 3 4 5
Understand family interactions	1 2 3 4 5
Manage strong affective expression	1 2 3 4 5
Assess the family using the GARF scale	1 2 3 4 5
Provide psychoeducation	1 2 3 4 5
Intervene in basic problems	1 2 3 4 5
Know when to refer complicated problems	1 2 3 4 5

B. Interview Behavior Checklist

The resident:

Engaged family members	Yes	No
Reviewed the structure and purpose of the evaluation	Yes	No
Obtained information about the referring doctor	Yes	No
Obtained identifying information about the current living arrangements	Yes	No
Obtained names and ages of children	Yes	No
Asked about others living in household	Yes	No
Asked about ethnicity/culture	Yes	No
Asked for each person's version of the presenting problem	Yes	No
Obtained the couple's history	Yes	No
Obtained an individual history from each	Yes	No
Obtained a three- or four-generation genogram	Yes	No
Identified significant issues of the family (e.g., job stress, birth of children, illness or death of significant people)	Yes	No
Inquired about substance abuse	Yes	No
Did the resident use language that was appropriate to both partners?	Yes	No
Did the resident ask at least one question about family strengths?	Yes	No
Did the resident allow or request an enactment?	Yes	No
Did the resident control the session appropriately (encourage both to speak, end arguments when appropriate)?	Yes	No

C. Family Therapy Competency Evaluation

Resident Year: 1st or 2nd (circle)

Rating Scale: Poor 1 2 3 4 5 Excellent (3 = expected level of performance)

General Competencies

Attendance/participation	1 2 3 4 5
Ability to use supervision	1 2 3 4 5
Overall clinical judgment	1 2 3 4 5

Specific Competencies

A. Cognitive/Conceptual Knowledge

1. Knowledge of family concepts and systems theory — 1 2 3 4 5
2. Understanding dimensions of family functioning using McMaster Model — 1 2 3 4 5
3. Recognize when family treatment is indicated — 1 2 3 4 5
4. Understand typical family transactional patterns — 1 2 3 4 5

B. Perceptual/Clinical Knowledge

1. Ability to engage the family in the assessment process — 1 2 3 4 5
2. Ability to identify transactional patterns — 1 2 3 4 5
3. Recognition of affect in family members and in therapist — 1 2 3 4 5

C. Executive Skills

1st Year:

1. Ability to do assessment and present problem list to family (minimum 3 assessments) — 1 2 3 4 5
2. Ability to work with the affect in the family — 1 2 3 4 5
3. Ability to pace work correctly to family's level of functioning — 1 2 3 4 5

2nd Year:

1. Ability to construct a treatment contract — 1 2 3 4 5
2. Ability to help family develop new, healthier transactional patterns — 1 2 3 4 5
3. Ability to know when and how to successfully terminate — 1 2 3 4 5
4. Ability to identify other treatment needs, if any, with the family — 1 2 3 4 5

14

Conclusions and Future Directions

The main goal of this manual is to provide a guide for the physician who is interested in involving families in the care of his or her patients. An additional goal is to encourage physicians, especially psychiatrists, to become more comfortable with including families in their treatment of psychiatric disorders. We have outlined an approach and a method designed to help clinicians to be able to evaluate the contribution of the family system to the presenting problems and to be able to help families, together with the patient, deal better with difficulties they are facing.

Many psychiatrists recognize that a focus on a narrow (often pharmacological) approach to the treatment of their patients' illnesses does not yield the level of results that they hope for or that are suggested by efficacy studies. Many trainees applying for positions in psychiatric residency programs increasingly look for programs that also prepare them to deal with psychosocial aspects of their future patients' lives. They recognize the importance of not abandoning the psychosocial foundations of the psychiatric profession. They are aware of the limitations of treatment approaches that focus too narrowly on attempts to control symptoms without also trying to help patients and their significant others cope more effectively with their illness.

We outline a clear and systematic model that allows a therapist to comprehensively evaluate the functioning of patients and families to facilitate a biopsychosocial formulation and treatment plan. A biopsychosocial formulation and plan address the primary illness as well as its impact on intrapsychic and interpersonal functioning. We emphasize that the key ingredients in approaching families have less to do with the personality style and unique skills of a particular therapist and more to do with adherence to a systematic format that ensures that there will be no major gaps in addressing the range of issues that could significantly influence the course and outcome of a patient's illness.

Not all families of psychiatric patients are dysfunctional. In fact, many families deal very effectively with recurrent, chronic, and severe illnesses. We emphasize the importance of recognizing and reinforcing resilience and competence. Even well-functioning families, however, can benefit from more information about an illness, validation of effective ways of coping, and reinforcement of resilience in the face of major stresses. Being clear about what constitutes functional or dysfunctional families or normal versus pathological ways of dealing with difficult situations is an important base from which to be able to make evaluations about the functionality of any family.

We place emphasis on the importance of a comprehensive assessment of the patient, the presenting illness, and the family context in which the illness exists and evolves. It is tempting for therapists to take shortcuts, to jump to conclusions, to focus on pet theories, or to avoid looking at too many aspects of patients' and families' lives for fear of finding problems that they may not want to deal with. It is self-evident, nonetheless, that effective treatment is most likely to follow comprehensive assessment. It is very difficult to develop an effective treatment plan without understanding the details of the clinical presentation, the individual's way of understanding his or her illness, ways of managing difficult situations, and the quality of support systems. A comprehensive assessment of the patient and his or her family allows the greatest opportunity to develop a treatment plan most likely to meet the needs of a particular family.

The extent of the assessment will, by necessity, vary somewhat depending on the clinical situation and the setting in which the assessment takes place. Although a comprehensive family assessment may be helpful for the management of acute psychiatric crisis in an emergency room, the acuity of the presenting problem, the sensitivity of the patient to too much stimulation, and the patient's inability to be in touch with reality may limit what can actually be done. We provide guidelines for the ways in which families can be engaged in the treatment process in a variety of clinical settings. The depth and breadth of family involvement may vary in different settings, but what should remain constant is the recognition of the importance of the family in any setting.

A central theme throughout this book is the importance of a biopsychosocial formulation. The biopsychosocial formulation has fallen out of favor over time because it is seen as simplistic or even irrelevant. There is an assumption that psychiatry has developed a more precise understanding of and ability to influence biological processes that are presumed to underlie major psychiatric illnesses. From our perspective, the biopsychosocial formulation's major value lies in reminding physicians to think broadly about the variety of forces that are involved in the pathogenesis, course, and response to treatment of the disorders that we are treating. The biopsychosocial framework reminds us to explore and understand the biological underpinnings of our patients' difficulties as well as the meaning that this illness has for them, their ways of coping with it, and the social environment in which the illnesses exist. At a minimum, we can help patients and families to better understand the nature of the difficulties they are struggling with, support them in dealing with these difficulties more effectively, and, most importantly, help families to change and function better.

Rational clinical decision making is likely to follow smoothly from a comprehensive biopsychosocial formulation. This formulation will make evident what the needs of the patient may be and what can or cannot be done to help. Therapists have to decide on the appropriateness of a family intervention, the timing of the intervention, and who is in the best position to provide care. There are a number of different models to help a physician decide the level of involvement he or she feels comfortable with in the management of patients and their families. Some physicians may choose to share the care of their patients with other mental health professionals. Other physicians may feel more comfortable providing comprehensive biopsychosocial treatments on their own. There is no absolutely right or wrong way to integrate biological, psychological, and social treatments. There are advantages and disadvantages to different approaches. Patient and family choice as to the number of therapists they wish involved should, of course, be a major part of that decision.

Every psychiatrist should be able to use family interventions. There are many schools of family/couples therapy and interventions but no evidence that any particular school is consistently superior to others. Multiple family approaches have been empirically tested, and many have been found to be useful for particular patient populations. Learning to do family therapy is not easy, and, like any other psychiatric intervention, requires practice. However, it is very difficult to become proficient using multiple models of family therapy. We have therefore taken the position that physicians interested in learning family therapy skills are best served by focusing on one or two models of therapy as opposed to borrowing bits and pieces from many models.

The model that we have chosen to use as the template for approaching families is the Problem-Centered Systems Therapy of the Family. This approach is predicated on a systematic process that includes the stages of orientation, assessment, formulation, treatment, and closure. The majority of families can benefit from the process of following these stages of treatment.

There are many ways in which family therapy/intervention skills can be acquired. We outline some useful approaches. It is unlikely that any physician or psychiatrist who is well established in his or her practice is going to find the time for training to become a proficient family/couples therapist. However, understanding the rationale for involving families encourages physicians to include families in the assessment and decision-making process about care. Psychiatric residents need to be exposed to the extensive literature showing the importance of family environment in the course of psychiatric illnesses and the effectiveness of family/couples interventions in improving treatment outcome. Psychiatric residents need supervision to become comfortable with family intervention skills through exposure and practice. Residents are also unlikely to start meeting with families unless they see that respected role models include families in their treatment. It is important for training programs to identify psychiatrists who are family oriented (as opposed to nonpsychiatrists) to supervise residents and act as mentors and role models.

There is great excitement in the field of psychiatry currently about the promise of functional neuroimaging and molecular genetics for the understanding of the etiology of many psychiatric illnesses. These fields carry the promise of targeted treatments that can deal effectively with the underlying pathophysiology of psychiatric disorders. At the same time there is a resurgence of interest in the broader psychosocial context of these illnesses. It is becoming clearer that there are significant gene-environment interactions that are manifest even in the short term. These interactions may be significant not just for the understanding of the etiology of a given disorder but also for the promise of how disorders can be managed over time. Disorders can be treated by attempting to manipulate receptors at the molecular level and also by shaping the broader social environment to influence receptor sensitivity and gene expression. It is this recognition and understanding of the complicated interplay between biological, psychological, and social forces that holds the most promise for the future of psychiatry.

Index

*Page numbers printed in **boldface** type refer to tables.*